If you are feeling overwhelmed, this book is your roadmap to healing your brain, and finding hope again – *Growth happens in the dirt.*

Testimonies

"I wish my wife had this book to read with me, it may have saved my marriage. But I do feel that it might save somebody else's - a guide for all people involved, meant to be read <u>together</u>.... This book needs to be part of every family who experience a TBI."

"After reading your 'message for the carer', for the first time my husband just held me and didn't try to fix me. I finally feel like he understands how I'm feeling".

*"Now I know what you and ***** went through, I'm sorry we weren't there for you, we didn't understand, but now we do".*

"What you say about a brain injury being an 'inside illness' is so true. I hope more people read this book to understand how it really feels."

"I found it hard to read the first part, because your story mirrored mine. But seeing the transformation gives me hope, my brain can heal".

"I never knew how important my brain was until I lost the use of it. It was the loneliest time of my life. I understand now how I have to care for myself every day".

Copyright Page

ISBN: [978-0-473-73911-9]
Publisher address: C/- NZ ISBN Agency Wellington 6144

First Edition

Growth Happens in the Dirt

Healing the Brain, Mind, and Spirit After Mild Traumatic Brain Injury

By Katie Jolly

A Journey Through Trauma, Recovery, and

the Science of Healing

Dedication

This book is dedicated to everyone in my life who journeyed out of the mud with me, and for you – the person reading this. I know how hard it can be and I want you to know that **you are not broken** – *the brain can heal*.

Thank you to my husband, the eye of the storm; my two beautiful children; my dad who saved my life with a random visit; and my mother who has taught me that to receive, we need to give. To the concussion team who taught me many of the skills that I share in this book. For Dr Daniel Amen and Tana Amen and the Amen Clinic, whose revolutionary work in brain health gave me hope. Thank you to the specialists Mark Grant, Colin Hancock, Vicki Gould, Bradley Pillay, Ryan O'Connor and Brenton Clark for generously sharing their knowledge to support those with concussion. To Mae Gomez, Philip Romano, Juliette George, Wendy O'Callaghan and Alison Sutton, Barbara Gustavson, Sonia Naea, Vicki Febery and Geoff Walker and my clients with concussion who helped me to craft this book. To my friends and brain gardeners' community, I am grateful beyond words.

Sir Isaac Newton, the famous English scientist, once said, 'If I have seen further, it is by standing on the shoulders of giants.' This book is built with a tribe – my healing journey has been the result of many helping hands.

From mess to message, supporting you with your brain health.

Keep shining x

Katie

Contents

A message for you, the concussion survivor

'The wound is where the light enters you,' Rumi

You are in the fight of your life for your brain, your sanity and your relationships. Being diagnosed with a brain injury is scary – not just for yourself but for everyone around you. It includes the ones who see who you 'were', as well as the rest of the world who don't understand why you've 'changed'. Or perhaps you say the wrong thing, or some days don't want to participate at all.

But trust me, my friend, you are going to **grow in the dirt**. It won't be easy, but it will be worth it.

Small trivial tasks that were once trivial may seem hard. Your moods may feel like a roller coaster and the biggest fear can be 'Will I ever be normal again?' Give yourself grace and quiet. Be kind to yourself on this journey and know your triggers.

The tools in this book are work that you implement daily – some of them are forever. But when you focus on healing your brain, you will find that a remarkable thing happens. You can start to function again. Wherever you are starting from right now, know that daily action is the secret sauce to succeed.

During this journey my marriage was in tatters. I couldn't parent and I lost many of my friends. I also lost my job and my identity and felt worthless to the point of darkness. Everything I knew that was 'me' was being ripped out in moments.

Some days I slept in the cupboard, some days I cried in the cupboard. Anger often overtook me and some days I sat with nothing in my head at all.

I walked into rooms not knowing why I was there, becoming so frustrated with the changes in my brain that I wanted to rip my head off.

Other days I would see people and couldn't converse, feeling naked, vulnerable and completely inadequate in the real world.

I've realised that a brain injury is an inside problem; those are the worst for others to understand. Like so many other illnesses that are on the inside, you don't get the same empathy because often there isn't visible evidence – like a broken bone. But just like a broken bone, the brain can get better. You will be different, but you can be more than you feel you are right now. **Growth happens in the dirt.**

You will be able to regain a quality of life once more, regulate your emotions and handle humans again. I see you, and you are kintsugi, a beautiful piece of art that can be glued together with gold.

From what I have since learnt about the brain, there is a part called the limbic system. Feeling safe is the major key in transformation. That is why you would rather stay in bed, or stay home when you feel unwell. It is why we gravitate to comfort (safety) foods or habits when we feel unwell. To grow in this journey, you need to feel safe. So take *small steps*, small steps that feel safe for you.

You may feel planted, but that is where seeds go to grow – in the dirt, and in the darkness. Underneath the soil you are going to heal. This is your time, and you deserve your place in the sun. Every day in every way you are getting better and better. It is time to give your brain the ultimate reverence it deserves.

Keep shining x

How to use this book

This book is designed to be a toolbox for you and your loved ones to support your concussion recovery. I couldn't read for seven months after my injury, so this work needs to be done together. If you are alone in your journey, I cannot stress enough how important it is to work with your medical provider during this time.

Medical disclaimer: The information provided in this book is intended for your general information. It is not a substitute for medical advice from a health care professional and is not intended to diagnose, treat, cure or prevent any disease. Always consult your doctor or other qualified health care professional with any questions you may have regarding a medical condition. Do not disregard medical advice or postpone consultation with your health care professional because of information that you have received.

My message is that 'mental health is brain health, and the brain can heal' due to my own struggles with anxiety, depression and ADHD for many years prior to the concussion. Yet when I focused my attention on healing the brain, I managed to successfully use these strategies to come off prescribed medications, including migraine, anti-depressants, nerve inhibitors and countless others.

In this I have been blessed by the collaboration of six specialists who have contributed to the resource section of the book. These sections are beneficial for practitioners who want to understand the dynamics and recovery of concussion more deeply. The contributors are:

1. **Mark Grant** is an Australian psychologist/researcher with 30 years of clinical experience. He has pioneered trauma-informed treatment of chronic pain and MUS with EMDR and lately hypnosis. Eye Movement Desensitization and Reprocessing (EMDR) is a psychotherapy treatment that is designed to alleviate the distress associated with traumatic memories. He co-authored two chapters regarding EMDR treatment of pain for the Oxford University Press *Handbook of EMDR* (2024).

2. **Vicki Gould** is an occupational therapist who specialises in concussion with over 20 years of experience.

3. **Brenton Clark** is a leading neuro optometrist in NZ with over 30 years' experience. He has also completed the OEPF Clinical Curriculum in Behavioural Optometry and

is a member of the Australian College of Behavioural Optometry (ACBO) and the Neuro-optometric Rehabilitation Association (NORA).

4. **Bradley Pillay** is a neuro optometrist in New Zealand, specialising in alternative eye healing for concussion.

5. **Colin Hancock** is a New Zealand and Australia-registered physiotherapist with 27 years' experience. His professional background in treating concussion injury started 12 years ago managing sports injuries sideline.

6. **Ryan O'Connor** is a neuro optometrist in New Zealand, who works with eye exercises for concussion recovery.

7. **Amen University** gave their permission for me to use authorised content from the Amen protocols for supporting change and mental health.

The chapters are built step by step as I worked through my journey, yet there is no right way to read this book as each section stands alone with a theme. I invite you to read the book for whatever you need now. Remember that change is like an unfolding lotus flower, you don't need to implement everything all at once: *build your health like you would a home.* Brick by brick. With any brain injury, it is important to build your habits as you would a house, laying one brick at a time. If you are unable to read for long periods of time, choose one section or, ideally, get a support person to read to you. After each story there are teaching points for concussion, then exercises that you can start to implement for your wellbeing.

You will see a ![brain icon] **icon wherever the tools begin**.

Be warned. When you start implementing the techniques in this book, you may feel nauseous. You may feel triggered, and you may feel tired. The idea of concussion recovery is: 'Just go to your ledge and then stop. But be consistent daily.' The exercises that make you feel the sickest are likely to be the ones that you need for rehabilitation. But success is not 'boom then bust'. Do the rehabilitation EVERY day until you hit the ledge then STOP. Your tolerance will grow as your brain heals. At the back of the book, specialists have generously contributed to the resource section, to help you and those travelling with you on the journey. There are links to websites and recommended books to help you. Even if you don't have access to services, within this book are tools you can begin to implement today.

It is time to heal. **Growth happens in the dirt!**

Two people who changed me

Dr Daniel Amen and his wife Tana Amen changed my life. Dr Amen is the world leader in brain health and the founder of the Amen clinics. They have developed scientifically proven pathways to heal the brain through lifestyle, supplements and nutritional changes. He has written multiple best-selling books on brain health. His wife Tana Amen, BSN (Bachelor of Science in Nursing), RN (Registered Nurse) is a *New York Times* best-selling author, health and fitness expert and vice-president of Amen Clinics. I discovered their extensive work after my initial rehabilitation when I read *The Brain Warrior's Way*. Not only did the information mirror what I had learned during my naturopathic study, it was woven together with science for brain health, with clear nutritional guidelines, lifestyle factors and supplementation to help the brain. The Amen research on how the brain can be healed, is an ongoing lifeline as I continue to study how *brain health is mental health*.

I have since qualified as an Elite licensed brain health trainer through the Amen University. In the resource section, you will learn some of the content they teach through the Amen clinics and in the many books Dr Amen and his team have published.

Introduction

If this book can provide you with even an ounce of hope, then it's worth it. Today I am grateful for my brain injury, the lessons and the struggle out of the mud.

Before the incident I was a qualified natural health practitioner for many years but had given up my passion to work in the family tourism business. My love of nutrition, exercise and mindfulness was swallowed up for three years in the corporate world of staff, systems and making money. Going from helping people to managing people didn't make my soul sing. I was a mother of two young children, but they spent a lot of time in front of the TV as I juggled work and home life. I was married, yet I spent more time looking at my husband's faults than appreciating his beauty. We had a nice home, food on the table, but my gratitude for the small things was masked with an incessant need for more.

I was like a duck on water, with the outward appearance of gliding through life but underneath the legs were frantically running in all directions. Before the head knock, I felt a sense of dis-ease in my life on an emotional level. All I prayed for was a 'break', which is what was delivered, levelling me beyond what I thought was possible. But just like a seed planted in the dirt, what grew out of that darkness was incredible.

My marriage, which was in tatters, is now a deep and loving connection. I am *grateful* that we didn't walk away from each other at the most broken point in our lives. My connection with others is deeper because I understand the depths of human suffering. My understanding of the brain and its importance has reframed my passion for health, because as I healed through lifestyle changes, I have eliminated countless medications.

Was any of this easy? No.

Was any moment of the journey without pain and struggle? No. To be brutally honest, the maze out of concussion is literally a battle of discipline. Yet when we make the work about our brain, amazing things can happen.

I still exercise daily; eat clean food; avoid negative information, people and situations that are damaging, all to be the bodyguard for my brain. Your mind is prime real estate, so create boundaries to protect your peace.

And the gift of going through a healing crisis is that when you are on the other side, you can then go back in and help others. I have more joy in my heart than ever before. The gift of *growing in the dirt* is that you won't be the same, but you can be *more* than you were before. You will be different, but you can heal. I am now fully immersed in natural medicine again concentrating on brain health, with the bonus of being a certified Dr Amen Elite Brain Health Trainer. Because I understand the struggles of not having a working brain, and the gift is to be able to help others out of the mud. If I hadn't banged my head, I would still be stuck on the corporate rat wheel. My head was damaged, but my heart was opened. As a result, I have moved back into my passion of helping others. Sometimes we are planted to get back to the roots of who we really are.

You may not be able to see it right now, but the mess can become your message. Many people who I have met who have experienced a brain injury are the kindest humans on the planet. They understand the depths of suffering, and have grown out of their own cocoon of darkness.

It is time to focus on you. Your healing. With the tools in this book, you can start to weave a beautiful carpet of wellbeing again. It will take time, and often there may be days when it feels you aren't making any progress, but just stick with it, and focus on consistency (not quantity).

Chapter 1

A message for you, the carer of someone with concussion (brain injury)

'Eventually you will come to understand that love heals everything, and love is all there is.' Gary Zukav

Dear loved ones

This is going to be tough, not only for the person that you love but also for you. **Read this book together.** It will give you an insight into what is happening and help you to avoid the pitfalls we made as a family.

What you need to understand is that the person going through concussion needs things from you that you have probably *never* given them before. Noise, light, too many people, too much talking, too many things in their day, will make them feel unwell. We call them *'triggers'* and that's what it is going to feel like some days, the feeling that someone has pulled the pin on an emotional grenade.

First and foremost, you need to realise that the anger, the tears and the words that come out of your loved one's mouth are not about you. If you can learn to not take anything personally, this journey will be easier. The biggest learning is to ignore the story (or the words) and listen for the emotion. When your person is crying because you've stirred the coffee anticlockwise, look for the *emotion*.

Their brain is hurting. Every task that was once easy is now confused and filled with headaches, rambling thoughts or no thoughts at all. When the brain is overloaded, it is like an electrical storm that will often rain on you.

Their amygdala (fight/flight/freeze/fawn) is overloaded right now, and one thing you can do to calm this is to make them feel safe.

The biggest healer is silence, and then physical touch. Love your person and realise a hug will say more than trying to get them to *explain* how they are feeling. Words don't heal a brain injury, but love will. Learn to hold tight to make them feel safe, because on many days they will feel lost, scared and out of control. When they move into *amygdala* mode, this is where the rage, tears, anxiety and numbness occur.

Don't ask if they need help, just do it. In the first months (depending on the severity of the injury), look at what you can do to ease pressure. If you're a parent and there are school drop-offs, do it; if there are errands, do them; if you can precook meals, do it. Anything to ease the daily pressure, because in the early stages your person needs quiet rehabilitation and will find daily life hard.

Your person is not your person for a little while. They are struggling with frustration that their mind is moving slowly, their body hurts, they can't find the words to make *you* feel better – so accept them where they are and love unconditionally.

The best moments of my recovery were when my dad would come out to the house and work. He would potter and do odd jobs and stop for a cup of tea. He was in my presence but didn't ask questions or talk much. He was just there. There is great healing in just being there for your loved one.

There will be days when your person is angry. Anger and frustration may fly at you. I regret wholeheartedly using my husband and my parents as punching bags, but the frustration with my brain was intense.

A powerful tool for you as a carer is to use the following method of communication:

1. Use empathy first – 'I'm sorry you seem angry/sore/tired.'
2. Then identify the emotion – 'You sound really angry. Why are you so angry? Are you angry with me?'
3. Give space and listen to allow them to unpack the emotion. Often this will bring it back to your beloved explaining that 'It's not you, it's just that I'm tired.'

When your loved one is losing their rag, don't leave the situation entirely. Go and take a few deep breaths outside, then re-enter. If you leave your loved one alone the dark emotions can start to escalate. Suicidal ideation is very common with concussion.

Hold tight but give space

So if your person is ranting/crying/spinning out of control, try this:

- Listen to the emotion, and then clarify 'You sound really _____ Is that right?'
- Ask them 'What's making you feel _____?'
- Ask them 'Do you need a hug, or space/sleep/time in the cupboard?'
- If they keep screaming at you, say 'Okay, I don't like this behaviour [this is key, as it's not the person, it is the

behaviour]. I'm going to give you some space and come back when you've calmed down.'

I've read books about brain injury that say 'You need to tell the person you won't be spoken to like that', etc, and that's fine. But in the heat of the moment, all those comments do is fuel the fire. Your person may not be emotionally conscious, almost like when you get drunk and something else takes over your body. *Treat your person like a toddler having a tantrum.* Don't lock them in their room as such, but do the identification process above and then suggest they have a rest. When they calm down after a brain break, talk to them about their words that you didn't like, so they can process what happened.

Your person loves you. Never ever forget that. The hardest thing you will deal with is that you can't *see* the injury. They just appear crazy. And they *are* crazy compared to who they were. But every day, inch by inch, bit by bit, your person will get better.

If you can go to sleep having settled differences, and in the morning treat it like a new day, then you will help your person immensely. This is what my husband did well. We went through nasty moments and every morning he would wake up and hug me and give me the opportunity to be better. *Holding onto hurt won't heal anyone.*

Every appointment that your person has (unless they ask you not to), please go. They will not remember what is said and every specialist I went to made me repeat my story again and again. If you can get time off, drive them to appointments. With a head injury the world suddenly becomes a scary place in which the normal they once knew has evaporated.

If you have children, include them in the rehabilitation process. Children need to understand if mum or dad or their sibling is dysregulated emotionally that *it is not their fault*, it is the broken brain that is to blame. This needs to happen early on, because there was no worse moment than one day seeing my children cower in fear in front of me because of my reaction to the fact that they were laughing too loud. Heartbreaking stuff.

If you are a parent, create a space for your children where they can just be kids, being mindful that too many competing noises will create overload for the person with a head injury. You may want to move the TV and stereo into another room, so that your person can cope with conversations in the family room. Multiple sources of sound can trigger concussion responses.

Your person will have peaks and troughs in their energy, which you need to be aware of. The best analogy came from one of the early specialists who explained:

'With a head injury your energy is like a pie. For a normal person, they can replenish their energy through rest, but for someone with a brain injury, once the pie is gone it is gone for the day. You need a full night's sleep to replenish the pie. So use your pie wisely.'

Early in the brain injury recovery your person's pie may be completely taken out by having a shower and making their bed or having a 10-minute conversation with someone about how they are feeling. When the pie is starting to run out for your person, you may see the following cues:

- Look at their eyes. You will see fatigue. They will possibly be struggling to keep them open, or they may be squinting (a sign that a headache is starting) or staring into space.
- They may start to get irritable with you or with things in general. This is a sign they are needing a brain break.
- They may start complaining about the noise, the light or the pain.
- Their words start to trip (this was my cue), they can't finish sentences, they switch words around, or they start to lose track of their conversation, talking about different things, rambling.

Each person will have a different set of triggers, but the faster you see signs and suggest for a brain break, the easier the recovery will be. Tell your loved one that you are in this together and you are there to support them.

In the beginning for most inside illnesses (the ones you can't see such as head injury, cancer, autoimmune, mental health) people are supportive. But as soon as a week later, people disappear and go on with their lives. You need to know this is not a short-term fix. Your person is going to need you there, and some days will be better than others, but in the first few months you are literally their lifeline to the outside world.

Don't try to drag them out socialising to cafes, restaurants or anywhere else where there is a lot of noise. This may make *you* feel better, but your beloved needs quiet.

If you have small children, sort the sleeping arrangements early on, as this was one of the major things that set me back. Night-creeping toddlers who disturb the sleep cycle are the worst for concussion recovery.

This is going to be hard – hard for you, but harder for the person you love who is struggling with post-concussion. Your person may be lost inside their own body right now, and they need time to heal.

For me, it was a grieving process. Grieving that the person that I was (a multitasker, corporate mother and a go-getter) had changed into someone who had very little joy in my heart at all. My brain changed and things that weren't hard (like making my bed and driving a car) were extremely taxing.

Let your person know you love them; it's an incredible anchor in this whole growth journey. If every day you wake up and decide that you are just going to love your person, you will get through this.

In life I've found that it's not so much what happens to us (the stories), as it is who we are with, and who is left at the end of the storm. *Your person needs you now more than ever, more than they will possibly ever need you again.* So weather this with them, you will get through it. **But know, that you also need support for you**. Look at creating your own tribe of people who can walk this path with you.

Lots of love to you and your family on this journey. It's hard. I've been there myself and then my son experienced post-concussion just a year after my injury. It is going to be hard . . . *but it's worth it.*

Chapter 2

The accident

'The tiny seed knew that in order to grow, it needed to be dropped in the dirt, covered in darkness and struggle to reach the light.' Sandra Kring

A TREASURE HUNT

It was Covid lockdown 2020. Our tourism business had been reduced from a staff of 35 to eight employees, including my husband and myself. Within three days, 95 per cent of our projected income was decimated as around the world borders closed with a violent bang.

We were stuck at home, frantically trying to juggle saving our business with schooling our children (a girl aged three and our son aged seven), and our marriage was beginning to fragment like winter leaves holed by frost.

Rotating duties like chicken in a supermarket oven, the husband and I would fight over whose turn it was to work on the business. At night we would watch the news as the world froze in fear. It was a fear that settled into our bones, as the children had nightmares about 'the virus'.

Stress was climbing into every part of our lives. My elderly parents were enclosed in their bubble, and we had only our family unit of four to rely on to create any resemblance of normality. Slowly, as the weeks passed, silence grew as my husband and I drowned in the fear of what would become of the business which was sliding through our fingers like dry sand.

My only solace was daily exercise with the kids. It was an opportunity to get outside in nature and feel a sense of freedom from the cage of Covid. 'Mum, can we do a treasure hunt tomorrow?' my seven-year-old begged. I looked at his pleading face, as his little three-year-old sister jumped on board with the idea. 'Yeah, Mama, a nature treasure hunt!'

I softened. 'Of course. Shall we draw up the map tonight before bedtime?' They both squealed with joy. It was always part of my game plan to wear them out as much as possible, so that I could work on the computer in the afternoon. It seemed perfect timing to have a picnic filled with at least an hour of bush running.

We sat in the lounge as they drew up the treasure hunt for the next day. Filled with local nature items, we planned an exciting expedition.

'Blackbird? Fern? Um, mushrooms? That's a good one, aye Mum!' as my son wrote the list on paper.

'Yep, that's great,' I smiled, seeing their eyes light up with the thought of a treasure hunt in the bush.

'Is Dad coming, Mama?" my little girl asked.

'No, babes, he's going to work.'

She lowered her blue eyes and then brightened. 'Can Brucie come?' (Brucie was the resident ADHD Chesapeake dog).

'Of course.' She smiled and gently slipped her thumb into her mouth, running her fingers along her 'frickie' (a satin hanky that was her comforter).

'I'll pack the picnic for tomorrow and we can spend the day in the bush,' I said. 'Come on then you two, into bed.'

As I tucked each of them in, my eyes filled with tears. Their little arms around my neck, glistening eyes filled with wonder . . . the sweet innocent sound of deepening breath as they fell asleep.

The monster Covid was at the door, but in that moment I had stopped being frightened. Everything seemed so fragile, and yet here in front of me was all that mattered. My babies, safe and warm.

The moment evaporated as I walked downstairs to start work again. I grunted at my husband who was sitting on the couch scrolling on his phone.

'Not sure when I'll be in bed,' I said, trying to make eye contact. 'I need to get this marketing stuff done before tomorrow.'

'Okay,' he grunted. He didn't even raise his head.

The one-word answers had become more frequent, silences filled with individual struggles of desperation. Both of us were finding it hard to be loving amongst the immense stress of losing everything we had built.

My eyes filled with tears as I fought the urge to collapse to the floor. 'No time for this shit,' I thought. Easier to just get angry at the husband and keep fighting forward.

So I turned on the computer and started running. That's all you can do, right? When a monster is chasing you – you keep running. Running fast from Covid-19, a monster we couldn't even see. Yet we were about to meet another monster worse than Covid . . . head on.

THE RUN THAT CHANGED MY LIFE

The next morning it was a stunning cloudless sky. Sun glistening on autumn leaves, with a light dew kissing the lawn.

As my husband started to leave for work, I stopped him and asked, 'What time are you finishing?' He whispered on the move, not making eye contact, 'Not sure, I'll be home when I'm done.'

My blood boiled quickly. 'Well, I need to do my work too!' Swiftly he was in the car, trying to avoid the inevitable conflict that was bubbling.

'The kids want to see you too!' I called back. Sunglasses on, he said nothing. The engine roared into life as the kids ran outside to hold my hands.

"Well, what's important right now?" I held back tears. He wound down the window, "Keeping our business afloat" he said flatly."I'll see you later, love you." The kids yelled "Love you, dad!"

As the truck roared away on the gravel road, I thought, 'What's important to me?'

When nothing is important, everything is important.

I bit back tears, the heaviness in my heart once more, and grabbed the backpack from the steps. 'Let's go and get busy before I fall apart, okay guys? Who's got the treasure map?'

They were so excited, as the dog jumped on the back of the truck. 'I do,' the tiniest replied, her chubby fingers tightly clutching the green paper. 'Who's got the picnic?' My son yelled 'Check!' 'Who's got the pens to mark the treasure off?' 'All good, Mum, let's go!' The dog was on the back, and we were in bush-bashing mode.

We pulled into the carpark and within minutes the game was on. The bush was deserted due to the Covid-19 lockdown – we had the entire track to ourselves. Rutted earth, native trees, big overarching pines, and plenty of autumn fairy house mushrooms to squash on our way. Total ecstasy for an ADHD household in the bush. Now when we play as a family, we play fast, faster and fastest, and with weeks of bush bashing during lockdown, we were fitness ninjas.

Car locked, we immediately started running on the track, crashing through spider webs that had laced themselves across the path in the night. The kids squealed, 'Got a mushroom, Mama! Quick, tick it off.' Fantails clicked and whistled in the trees, the lake gently lapping in the distance.

Run, run, run – four hairy brown legs and six human legs – as fast as they could. 'Moth, Mama! Tick it off!' The pace was furious. By the time I'd marked it down, they'd disappeared again.

I lost sight of them for a moment and ran harder to try and catch up. 'What's the next one?' I screamed as the children ran ahead laughing. 'Mum, find a fern!' They disappeared into the distance followed close by Bruce the dog.

I felt so alive. My breath was deep and fast, and as the sun dappled the green leaves, I felt whole. Happy and connected with my kids at a time when the world was frozen in fear by a virus. I sprinted to try and catch up. With no humans in sight, I still needed the comfort of knowing my babies were not alone. A little bird flitted tree to tree beside me. Maybe I should have listened and slowed down.

I caught sight of them as I rounded the bend. **Then it happened**.

From that point on, all I remember was my right foot hitting a rock. The world felt as though it was in slow motion – the feeling you have in dreams when your feet lift from the earth, and you hover above the ground for several minutes. A kaleidoscope of fractured seconds, before gravity deals a heavy hand. As surreal as the memory is, in the next moment it shattered into pain as I fell to the ground hard.

Three rocks: one to trip on, one to smash my knee on, and the last crushed into my head. I had pushed my son over in the fall, and somewhere ahead on the track I could hear him screaming. But my whole body was unable to move.

I lay frozen on the soft earth moaning. My right leg seared with hot pain, while underneath my left temple was cold hard stone. My son was still screaming at the top of his lungs. Pavarotti (my son's nickname for his vocal ability) was in full swing, and my body was like stone.

'Noooooooo,' I moaned repeatedly, as pain radiated through every cell in my body. I slowly moved my head to see how far away he was from me.

My daughter crouched nearby sobbing. 'Mama . . . Mama.' I tried to move but couldn't; my leg felt broken.

Exhaling, I lay stuck like a monkey doing breaststroke in a mud river. I could feel a thumping pain in my shin, and cold rock pressed underneath. My left temple resting on another rock, eyes muddied with tears, the sound of my son sobbing, needing my help. 'Mama, are you okay? Mama! Mama!', the three-year-old's voice becoming more and more desperate.

I have no idea how long I lay there with the children by my side, or any recollection of the next six hours of my life, but somehow I got up.

A broken memory erased. The only rationale is that a will stronger than my own took over. The need to look after my children isolated any damage in my body and would continue to motivate me through the ordeal to come.

At least 50 photos in my phone of the adventure I couldn't remember. A video of the nature hunt and a 20-minute drive home completely erased from my memory. Life was about to change dramatically.

THE UNRAVELLING

That evening my shin felt broken and the pounding pain in my head was so intense that I felt as if I was floating above my body. The children recounted to my husband how I'd tripped on a rock, my leg landed on another rock and hit my head on a third rock.

'Are you okay?' he asked, concerned. 'Sure, I'm fine,' I snipped. 'Okay, well we're tenting out tonight in the gully,' he said casually.

I asked him to stay inside because I didn't feel well, but he had promised to sleep in the tent with our son. Maybe I didn't fully communicate how bad I felt, or maybe weeks of Covid lockdown had numbed his concern for me, so he went to the gully with my son, and I was left alone with our daughter.

Sore, vulnerable, feeling unloved, I lay curled up on the couch with my little girl as fat tears of pain streaked down my cheeks. Her three-year-old body nestled beside me as my head pounded. I had never felt so alone before, like a person stuck inside a snow globe where sound is muffled.

'Don't cry, Mama, it will be okay' as her tiny fingers wiped my cheeks. She whispered, 'I know it's sore, but if you take a deep breath, it will be better in the morning. I love you . . . Thank you, my babes,' as my eyes seared in pain.

But things would not be better in the morning. They would not be better for a very long time.

The next day it felt as if a veil had been placed over my head like a warm haze. My left eye had blackened, and although that concerned me, the leg was more of an issue. I couldn't bear weight, with each step a searing nail.

But I'm like any mama, right? We get up, we carry on, we don't complain, and we do what we must do. There wasn't time to feel sorry for myself – our business needed me. 'Do you need to go to a doctor?' my husband asked. 'Nah I'll be fine,' I replied, and so he went back to his routine.

My determined nature overrode the pain; with the kids on my own and work to do, there was no time for self-pity. Although I was aware that things were jarring, I ignored everything. Juggling the computer, pressures of homeschooling, activities, DIY around the house, it felt as if I was living in a psychedelic movie.

Yet just a few days after the incident, the symptoms were intensifying. The immense pain in my skull and leg were constant. For the first time in my life, I had insomnia – awake all night, eating toast on the coach, as if I'd had 60 coffees and somebody had switched the lights on in my head. I could hardly walk, my eye was swollen and blackened, and suddenly noise and light were a 'thing'. But because I knew nothing about concussion, I decided to dose up on painkillers, migraine pills (as I had suffered from them in the past), caffeine and my ADHD medication, and carried on working.

With the lack of sleep and increasing sensitivity to all stimulus, I became more aggressive with my family. When people suggested going to the doctor (because we were still in lockdown) I'd brush it off. I started to notice strange symptoms, with one eye closing slower like a magnetic hinged door. Waking up from a brief sleep, I would try to open and close the left eye but it would be on delay mode.

Walking down the stairs my whole body was tipped to the right. My head felt as if a knife was being driven into my skull.

Breakfast was migraine medication with a big cup of coffee – the kids in front of the TV and the rat wheel beginning again.

With the stress of Covid and the new symptoms, I began to fall into emotional overwhelm. It was as if everyone was conspiring against me with their noise. A pot of boiling rage sat within: the cutlery being put away, the children laughing, the headaches that violently radiated from the back of my neck, the aching shin. More painkillers, more coffee, more and more medication needed to function – but I carried on. Covid was the enemy and *I really thought everything I was experiencing was stress.*

Over the next two weeks my health and relationships deteriorated. I had no idea I was digging myself a bigger hole – personally and professionally. I felt lost in a sea of strange symptoms, slowly losing grip on reality. No sleep, constant pain, I was existing in an altered universe that was ripping me from those I loved. I'd sit on the stairs with my children's little arms wrapped around me crying 'It's okay, Mama, it's okay.' My parents were aware of the accident but could not visit due to the Covid isolation rules. Eventually my husband and I stopped talking. Three weeks after the accident the Prime Minister announced that restrictions were lifting and the children could return to school. The bubbles had popped, and life was to resume for everyone. Everyone except me. My bubble was about to pop big time. I had been planted in the dirt.

Get checked immediately

I *didn't* go to a doctor after the accident, and people have asked me why? Firstly, I didn't understand concussion, and my knee was in more pain at that moment, taking focus from the blurred vision or the headaches. I have had multiple head injuries during my lifetime, falling into a brick wall at four years old which split my eyebrow, a fall from a tall tree onto a concrete slab which knocked me out, and a slip on a parapet floor that left me in a neck brace for six weeks.

But on all those occasions, although my mood was unstable and the pain intense, I and those around me (including doctors) had no knowledge of the full effect of concussion. As a naturopath, we never studied the brain, let alone the impact of compound concussions on brain health. I had no idea of the impact a concussion could have on the brain, as I had never learnt anything on head injuries during my study. I didn't understand brain injuries, or even the notion that post-concussion was a 'thing'.

From years of boxing and intense sport, my tolerance for pain was high, and somewhere in the back of my mind I was downplaying the symptoms I was experiencing. Yes, I was in pain and my mood was sliding downwards, but I didn't have any blood (apart from my black eye the next day) so I felt that I could keep going. Ignorance escalated and prolonged my healing.

My mindset was to 'keep doing' so I tanked up on painkillers, ADHD meds and caffeine to keep the brain active. Secondly, our business was crumbling because of Covid, and with little time to sit around and feel sorry for myself, so I ignored my pain and sank my teeth into work.

Many of the psychological symptoms with concussion can mirror stress, and to say we were 'stressed' is a light statement. There were so many holes in my knowledge that I put up with the increasing symptoms until crisis point.

When I did contact the doctor after my mental health snapped (and it was during Covid, so all consultations were remote), he referred me to a local physiotherapist who specialised in concussion. At the time in our town, few doctors understood concussion, so the protocol was to outsource to a specialist team. From Colin Hancock, the concussion physio specialist, I was referred to the concussion team. In hindsight, I should have gone to the hospital immediately, yet as you will see in this story, we all *live* and then *learn*.

A concussion is an injury from a direct blow to the head, neck or face, or a force directed somewhere else on the body that transfers the force to the head. Symptoms can occur immediately or may evolve *over time.*

Any type of head knock should be *immediately* checked out. You do not have to have a 'black out' or have cracked your skull to have caused damage to your brain. The brain is like a ball of soft butter set into a case with spiny ridges, so any large impact to the head can cause concussion. Also, repetitive head knocks over time can cause brain injury (such as contact sports, falls) and may extend your recovery time.

Only 5 to 10 per cent of concussions result in a loss of consciousness.

Know who your team is

It is very easy when faced with adversity to forget that your family is your *team.* In sport, attacking the players of your 'team' makes no sense, and yet we often claw at those closest to us. Rather than banding together, we fall apart and use each other as the landing pad. As you move through your healing journey, *know your team.* They will be the ones who are there through the worst of your days and hopefully will still be standing beside you as you heal.

Stress

Stress is an interesting mistress. When you are recovering from concussion, all your emotions tend to be heightened. The brain resorts to its most primal instinct of 'fight, flight or freeze'. During periods of intense stress your immune system is weakened, so you are more likely to be sick. Your digestion is impaired, as your blood flow is shunted away from the gut to your limbs to prepare you for action. This is why a brain injury can mirror many other mental health disorders such as stress. You may be experiencing anxiety, depression, mood swings, rages – all of which align with a brain feeling fried. With concussion, the normal everyday moods are hit with radioactivity and feel like triple the 'normal' response. When you are 'stressed' the blood flow to your brain decreases.

You may experience:

- Increased heart rate
- Breathing high into your shoulders
- Inability to think clearly
- Mood swings

We feel unsafe, so the amygdala fires. When we feel stressed, the amygdala fires. You will fight, flee, freeze or fawn (I like to say fall in a heap), but overwhelm with concussion happens a lot faster than ordinary stress because our tolerance is depleted.

Using calming techniques regularly while you are healing can help you to self-regulate emotions. The most important tool for concussion recovery (or stress) is to learn how to calm down and take a BRAIN BATH.

Ideas for brain bathing:

- Sit in a dark cupboard with noise-cancelling earphones and focus on breathing in for a count of four, hold for a count of four, and breathe out for a count of four. Breathe deep into your belly until you feel calm again. Do this for a minimum of five minutes.
- Listen to a binaural beats track – the audio helps the brain to relax.
- Eye palming – rub your hands together for 30 seconds, then place over your eyes for a minute.
- Take a warm shower for five minutes.
- Look at a photo of something you love (or somewhere) for two minutes until your breathing regulates.
- Go for a walk outside in nature and whilst you are walking, breathe deep into your belly. Notice the sounds, sights, smells, and sensations. Wear a cap and sunglasses and even ear plugs to avoid over stimulation.

Just like gardening, in order to heal we need to:

Weed: external stimulation (noise, screens, people)

| Feed: | deep belly breathing, calming music, change environment |
| Seed: | take regular brain baths during the day |

🧠 *Every day change your environment twice*

During the concussion recovery you may want to stay inside all the time. Yet a powerful tool for mental health is to change your environment at least twice during the day. It is important to get Vitamin D (via sunlight) to help your brain to function well. Rolling up your sleeves and getting 10 minutes of sunlight onto your forearms will help with Vitamin D levels. If you are going for a walk (or sitting outside) in the first stages of your journey, ensure you:

1. Wear a peaked cap
2. Use noise-cancelling headphones or silicone ear plugs
3. Wear sunglasses
4. Set a timer for 10 minutes if the light is too much for you.

🧠 *Concussion symptoms*

With head injuries, you may not 'know' that you have hurt your brain. I boxed for a few years (only one fight to claim) and had previous falls, as I've described, yet apart from the muscle soreness, before this time I did not understand how fragile the brain is, nor the symptoms or major effects that concussion can have long term. If you've had a major accident, you will already know that your brain has been compromised. As I said earlier, you don't have to experience 'black out' to suffer a brain injury.

However, if you're a sports enthusiast or have had a knock to the head which didn't leave you in the hospital or blacked out, there are very clear signs to watch out for. Always take a head injury seriously. If you have any of these symptoms, get medical attention immediately:

- Sensitivity to light and noise
- Headaches and pressure behind the eyes or in the skull
- Brain fog and memory loss
- Insomnia (sudden onset meaning it hasn't happened before)
- Mood changes
- Speech or body movement changes
- Numbness or tingling (can involve the neck)
- Irrational behaviours (spending more money, poor decision making, etc)
- Concentration issues
- Balance issues
- Hearing changes or loss including ringing or buzzing
- Vision changes

Especially for parents whose children have had a fall or injury due to sport, it is vitally important to rule out brain involvement.

If you are experiencing these issues, see your doctor immediately and ask to be reviewed for post-concussion. There are specialists who deal with concussion that can perform assessments.

Migraine

A migraine is more than a bad headache. It can cause debilitating throbbing in one part of your head that can leave you in bed for days. Triggers can be:

- Movement (if there are structural issues in your neck)
- Bright lights or sunlight
- Sound
- Hormonal changes
- Dehydration
- Low blood sugar

Migraines may have pre-symptoms before they arrive:

- Seeing 'auras' which may appear as bright flashing lights, dark spots, or swimming vision
- Sensitivity to smells

- Strange sensations like crawling on the skin
- Nausea

An ocular migraine (ocular meaning 'eye') may involve losing vision or partial vision in one eye with the associated pain.

Migraines are a common side effect of a concussion. When you have a migraine, the following may help:

1. Lie in a dark room
2. Use an icepack on your neck or on the top of your head
3. Drink a glass of water with a pinch of Himalayan salt (especially if you suffer from low blood pressure)
4. Eat some sort of protein and fat (if the migraine is associated with hunger or low blood sugars); walnuts (containing Omega 3) have been shown to help with a migraine
5. Go for a walk in the fresh air (if you have been sedentary)
6. Place lavender oil on your wrist and inhale the smell

THE WATERMARK THAT BROKE THE CAMEL'S BACK

On the morning of 'freedom' post lockdown, as the country wound into work again, my husband drove away with the children in his truck. I was ecstatic. I could finally get some work done in peace! A breakfast of painkillers and coffee acidified my gut as I sat down to the laptop to do 'work'.

I was typing a sensitive document, when suddenly I hit a speed bump. I wanted to insert a draft watermark, but for the life of me I could not remember the word or even how to find what I needed.

My brain was blank. No matter how hard I tried, it felt like squeezing blood out of stone and I sat there for 20 minutes staring at the screen. Eyes burning, I started to type – my fingers were pushing all the wrong buttons. I couldn't type. My brain could see the words and what they should be, but my fingers wouldn't comply. Suddenly my breathing got rapid, ears numb, heart beating as though it would leap out of my mouth. As the pressure built like a steam engine train up a steep hill, I burst into tears and screamed like a wild woman for what seemed like an eternity.

Then suddenly something inside me snapped. Like turning off a light switch, all the emotion was gone, and an eerie clarity entered my mind.

'I must leave – right now – it is time to go! My family don't need me – nothing is important any more. Nobody needs me. The only solution is to go. I need to buy a tent and move into

the bush, leaving my family who will all be better off without me.'

With a rush of adrenalin, I took immediate action. It all made sense. Why had I not seen it this way before? With military precision, I ordered a tent online to pick up that day, then I ran around the house like a crazy woman packing everything I needed for my new life: medication, coffee, a sleeping bag, pillow, a few clothes and my yoga mat. Here I was in May (where zero temperatures were looming in the New Zealand winter), about to leave my home to live in a tent. No food or other supplies, just armed with a new life purpose that had overtaken me.

In under 30 minutes, I was packed to go. I thumped down into the driver's seat and turned the engine on. Blind with determination and no rational brain function at all, I didn't even notice that my father's car was entering our driveway. He parked alongside me with a quizzical look on his face. Dressed in his painter's overalls, he seemed like a mirage.

I had not seen him for two months because of the lockdown restrictions. He tapped on the window of my truck, pointing to the pile of my 'new' life and said, 'What are you doing?'

I blinked. His face was like a dream. My eyes darting nervously, I wound down the window with hands firmly on the steering wheel, stating 'I'm leaving the family, Dad, and going to live in the bush. I've had enough.'

His face furrowed in concern. 'What do you mean you're leaving?'

My eyes darted back and forth, my wonderful idea now sounded a little strange, and my grip on reality felt wobbly. Whether it was the first time I felt as if someone had 'heard' my pain or whether it was seeing my father, whom I adore with all my heart, I burst into a cascade of violent tears.

"Get out of the car and come inside,' and as his wiry arms wrapped around me, I felt swallowed up into the ground. All the ambition was drained from my bones, leaving me scared and vulnerable. I collapsed onto the couch and sobbed relentlessly like a torrent sweeping over a waterfall into a dark eddy, my body racked with sadness as I spun out of control. My dad just being there loving me had popped the cork on the emotional champagne bottle.

Whatever had been holding me together snapped, and my father witnessed the unravelling first-hand. 'What's all this?' He looked stunned, as if he'd walked into another country. We had been calling each other on Facetime, but conversation always centred on the kids' positive titbits, so my parents didn't know the full extent of our emotional upheaval.

Through the wailing discourse I cried 'I'm either going completely crazy or I've got a concussion. I just thought if I moved into the bush, everyone would be better off without me. I don't know what's happening, Dad . . . I'm going mad!'

Dad shook his head. 'Kate, get to the doctor. I can see you are not well – get this sorted now.' His pale face filled with love as I shook with tears.

'Where's Simon?' Dad whispered. 'At work,' I sobbed.

'Does he know how you're feeling?" He frowned. I whispered, 'We've been fighting.'

'Where are the kids?' he said, shaking his head. I wailed as snot poured down my nose into my mouth. 'School and day care. Simon is picking them up later.'

Dad blew out three little breaths, his default for when he's stressed. 'Get upstairs and call the doctor now, I'm not going anywhere until you do.'

Don't make life decisions right now

Do NOT make any major life decisions throughout your concussion journey, especially in the first stages of rehabilitation. Quite often the prefrontal cortex (the decision maker of the brain) goes offline, and we are ruled by our emotional body. It is vitally important to discuss any life changes with the people closest to you.

Find at least one person who 'sees' you and that you feel safe with; it is very easy to feel crazy in the beginning. This person should be able to hold space for you without necessarily having to 'fix' you. They can be a sounding board for your thoughts.

Please understand that your brain is not working properly now. An inspiration to sell your home, leave your relationship or purchase something may be the result of scrambled pathways. *Park all big decisions for at least six months after your initial accident.*

For those supporting someone with concussion, it is useful to just *be* with your person. Not talk, but just sit quietly and listen, to allow them to process what is happening inside their internal cage.

Chapter 3

The diagnosis

'The first step toward change is awareness. The second step is acceptance.' Nathaniel Branden

My balance was unsteady as I climbed our stairs to make the call in private. As the receptionist answered the phone, I explained the story which would become my swan song for months to come of 'tripping on a rock, leg hitting a rock, then left temple smashing against another rock'. Typical of Covid times, I was told the doctor would 'Call me back', and luckily he did so within minutes. He asked about my symptoms: light sensitivity (check), noise intolerance (check), insomnia (check) ('I'll prescribe some sleeping pills to help'), headaches and memory issues (check).

With a phone diagnosis of 'concussion', I was instructed to immediately go to the specialist in town to get assessed. I laughed on the phone. 'If it's not concussion, where do I go for a strait jacket, as I could really enjoy a paid holiday away from my humans at the moment.'

Dad hugged me as I got into the truck to travel the 15 minutes into the concussion physiotherapist's office in town. 'You'll be okay, babes. We'll look after you – be safe.'

It was the very first time I had driven into town for over six weeks, and it being the first day that humans were allowed out to resume 'normal' life the roads were busy. As I drove along the country road, head pounding and the world spinning, the white lines on the road seemed to sit far to the right, so I kept correcting myself.

Suddenly a car came screaming round the bend, parping it's horn to move me onto my side of the road. I realised that my eyes were playing tricks on me – right wasn't right at all, my driving was swanning over the midline.

Every car seemed like 10,000 of them coming at me. I couldn't judge how fast they were travelling and didn't know when to turn into the traffic. The truck crawled up the road under the speed limit, cars overtook me, people beeped their horns, and my heart felt as though it throbbed inside my throat. As I sat at the intersection, I couldn't judge when to move the car. Vehicle after vehicle lined up behind me, I just couldn't tell how fast things were going. All I could see was a blur of speed, hear my pounding pulse, and feel the sweat pouring out of my hands on the steering wheel. A loud toot, and I finally pulled out into the traffic to arrive at the specialist's office. Overwhelmed and fraught with anxiety, from a meagre 15-minute car journey.

🧠 *Can you actually drive your car?*

When you have a concussion, there are a few things that you must pay attention to. Firstly, your neck and your eyes. Quite often with a head knock your brain perceives vision differently. We need both our neck and our eyes to drive:

1. The eyes perceive not only oncoming cars, but the depth and speed of how fast they are travelling. You are required to look in many different directions to drive and be aware of many stimuli.

2. Your neck is required to look from side to side to check traffic, and if you are suffering from post-concussion, this small movement alone can make you feel nauseous.

If your brain injury has left you feeling nauseous when you change eye movement or move your head, you may need to consider stopping driving until you get assessed by a neuro-optometrist. Also the constant motion and scanning of your eyes can induce headaches.

On a sensory level, driving can make a person with concussion very symptomatic. Brain changes can create altered perceptions of distance and balance in the eyes. Your safety and the safety of others is important. If driving is triggering you, get your eyes checked as this can be a game changer for your symptoms.

In the beginning, you may find that travelling in a car even as a passenger makes you feel sick. It is very similar to 'sea sickness' due to your brain being tipped sideways. Depending on what part of the brain has been affected (or even your ear salts), keep car travel to a minimum, and always wear your sunglasses and a cap to avoid flashing lights on your peripheral vision.

THE CONCUSSION PHYSIO

As I arrived at the concussion physiotherapist's office, I parked the truck haphazardly (totally wonky in the lines). As I walked inside, a vibrant 'Hello!' from the over-enthusiastic receptionist immediately irritated me. She was too loud, the lights in the pale office were too bright, and as I tried to sit down the chair seemed off balance.

So I sat on the floor, literally flopped on the floor. Eyeballs burning like I was drunk at a nightclub. The receptionist appeared unphased by the tall blonde woman languishing on the carpet. 'Okay, you hit your head, so it will be an *accident* claim. Can you fill out the forms please', handing me the clipboard and pen.

My hand was shaking, I couldn't grip the pen properly, and the level of irritation was moving from zero to explosive in a few seconds. I couldn't remember my address, my phone number, the date – every thought felt excruciatingly hard, as I clawed for memories that just weren't there. I started to sweat and chew the inside of my mouth.

The receptionist saw my discomfort and gracefully walked to my spot on the carpet, gently extracting the greasy pen and clipboard from my hands. 'Don't worry, we will get this sorted for you. Do you have a contact number for your husband?' I handed her my phone.

As I was ushered into the sterile white room for the assessment, I felt scared. Scared that I would be labelled crazy, that I was making all of this up and the stress of Covid had flipped my sanity switch. The concussion specialist, a middle-aged balding man in a crisp polo shirt, eyed my notes and then placed the clipboard down. 'What happened, Mrs Jolly?' Again, the story of three rocks recounted.

He asked me if I had ever had a head injury before. I had experienced quite a few, as I described earlier. Once in my 30s I slipped on a hard floor and ended up in a neck brace for six weeks, as I've mentioned. Plus a few years of sparring without head gear during boxing training . . .

His demeanour immediately soothed away my anxiety, he was speaking softly and slowly. I felt as though I was in a place where I *may* be safe. 'Well, let's have a look at what's going on, shall we? I'd like you to remember these four words, and then we will do some testing for a few minutes. Then I will ask you to repeat them again – is that okay?' Four words, that sounded like an easy task! He then tested my eye movement and my balance and then asked me to repeat the original words. I couldn't.

'Okay, Katie, try counting backwards for me in twos.' I couldn't. He smiled gently. 'Okay, let's try . . .' but suddenly a wave of nausea crashed out of me like a tsunami. I screamed, 'I feel like I'm going to throw up!'

The session ended with a firm diagnosis of 'Mrs Jolly, you've got concussion, but how about you come back again to do further testing to see how bad it actually is.'

I drove home, rattled. It was like breaking a prize vase in a boutique store and not knowing the cost. I was entering unknown territory, a diagnosis without understanding what was happening to me.

That week the next two sessions at the concussion physio's office were even worse. I had to walk on a white line on the carpet, eyes open, to check my balance. All I had to do was stay on the line. My competitive spirit whispered 'You've got this one, easy as!' I walked that line with the grace of a broken-legged duck. I was appalled to find out that the average time was 14 seconds to complete the drill – I had taken one minute 24 seconds.

The physio smiled. 'How about we try balancing with your eyes shut now?' I fell over.

The final test was next door in the gym to monitor the brain under exertion. A serious fitness bunny, I laughed at the prospect of even feeling sick while exercising. '*It will take me a hell of a lot of hill climbs to make me hurl,*' my ego yelled. But as the treadmill started to move, the incline increased and the fluorescent lights of the gym pulsed in time with the Black-Eyed Peas, the walls were about to be decorated with my lunch! Getting irritated and hot, I felt as if I was going to faint. After just a minute, my bravado was obliterated and I needed to get off the treadmill before I exploded.

'Get me off, get me off – I'm going to be sick!'

Back in the physio's office I felt as if I was in a surrealist art film. The bright lights, the dulcet tones of the specialist, the pounding blood in my head muffled the words. 'Mrs Jolly, you have suffered a mild TBI, a Traumatic Brain Injury. I'm going to put the referral through to the concussion programme immediately. You must come off all caffeine, alcohol and screen time straight away. You need to stop work immediately and I would suggest that you stop driving until we can get you assessed further. I will put this through as an urgent request for the concussion team.'

'Can I get something to help with my sleep? I haven't slept in days.'

'Your doctor can prescribe you something for that.'

As I drove home, head swimming from nausea, I mulled over the words. '*Mild TBI*' – that doesn't sound that bad. *Mild*. Mild! Mild traumatic brain injury. **Mild!!** That sounded like a week recovery tops! Little did I know that 'mild', like most things, is a sliding scale, and this was only the beginning of the journey.

Compound concussions

It is important when you see the specialist to mention any previous concussions, or whether you have played a contact sport in the past that may affect your healing. Many accumulated knocks over the course of time can affect your brain health.

If you're a parent of children who play contact sport, be aware that head injuries are accumulative. If you notice any changes in personality, or your child complains of headaches, nausea or behavioural issues at school, you will benefit from seeing a concussion specialist to assess their brain health.

Get an advocate early on

When you have ANY appointments during the first stages of concussion, always take someone with you. That person needs to be your driver and can voice any concerns that you may not be noticing at the time. If you are unable to fill in forms, this person can do these for you. There is a real risk if you don't have an advocate. Due to stress you will miss vital information that will help you in the long term.

Depending on the level of your brain injury, you may or may not already have an advocate. Why do you need one?

- You may be under stress visiting doctors and specialists and the environment will cause your brain to malfunction
- You may not be able to articulate your needs well
- You may not remember what has been said
- You may not be heard and therefore not get the care you need
- Your memory may be impaired and miss communicating vital information that the specialists need to tailor your care

🧠 *What to do before any specialist appointment*

Be prepared before you see the doctor, physio or any specialist. Prior to the appointment get your support person to take notes of all current symptoms:

- Is your medication working / not working / are there any side effects?
- Are there any new symptoms developing?
- How is your sleep and mood?
- Has there been any change in your pain (increase or decrease)?

Often a specialist's office will have fluorescent lights and noise, which can trigger symptoms. This may affect your brain function during the appointment. Wear a peaked cap, and in the waiting room wear sunglasses if needed.

Write down a list of questions before the appointment, as often with the medical system there will be no access outside of this time. Take your questions with you to get answered during the session.

Ask your advocate to take notes, and if you can't articulate how you are feeling, allow your advocate to speak for you.

You may have to grant permission for your advocate to act on your behalf if dealing with government organisations. If you are entitled to any benefits or additional support, having a person helping to navigate the government organisations will be helpful.

Always review your medication if it is not working for you, or if any symptoms are not improving and worsening.

Testing for concussion

Please be aware that your local doctor may not be trained in concussion. Having a brief balance test is not enough. If you are still symptomatic, it is vital that you receive an assessment from a specialist who is trained in head injuries.

Concussion screening tools check the brain's processing and thinking function after a head injury. They measure physical skills such as balance but also mental skills such as memory, concentration, attention and how quickly you can think and solve problems.

Depending on where you get assessed they may also look at:

- How your eyes are moving
- Your ear salts (which can become unbalanced, causing vertigo)
- Your neck function (most head injuries also involved whiplash)

- If you can reverse information (like saying the months backwards or subtracting numbers)
- Your history of concussion, and any other issues such as ADHD, mental health issues
- The severity of concussion symptoms (headache, nausea, sensory issues, etc) and whether there are any urgent issues like developing seizures, numbness, or weakness in the body.

If you are at home, and your loved one has suffered a head injury, there are some basic tests that you can perform to confirm whether concussion may be an issue:

- Do they feel dizzy, nauseous or have a headache?
- Ask them to track your finger with both of their eyes. Draw a large 'X' with your finger and see if they can follow with both eyes.
- Is there any slurring of speech?
- Is one pupil larger than the other?
- Is your person sensitive to light, sound, or movement at all? They may suddenly develop travel sickness in the car.
- Has there been a sudden change in behaviour? More aggression, anxiety or confusion?

- Ask them to repeat a basic sequence backwards (10 - 0) or remember a birthday or another important date that normally they would know.

Medical diagnostics

There are several diagnostic tools that you will go through to diagnose your brain injury. From simple balance exercises and memory to psychological testing, you need to understand what the bigger ones do, so that you can push for further assessment if you are not getting better. Understanding what the tests are can help:

1. An x-ray will see broken bones.
2. A CT scan can detect blood clots, muscle damage, cancers; it reveals dysfunction or change of structure in bone, muscles and organs.
3. An MRI uses strong magnetic fields to take pictures of the inside of the body. It is more detailed than a CT scan but will often not show brain damage (unless the trauma is severe).
4. A SPECT scan (which the Amen Clinics use) show what areas of the brain are more active or less active to provide a comprehensive overview of damage to the brain.

🧠 *Medical support*

If you have a serious concussion, you will need to consider the following:

- Medication to help with pain management, mood regulation and brain function
- Manual therapy to help with pain management
- Specialised neuro optometry to rebalance your brain
- Neuro physiotherapy
- Counselling
- Occupational therapy

If you find that the medication or therapy is not helping you, let your specialist know. These things are designed to support you, and if they are not working inform your medical team.

🧠 *Must-have accessories*

As soon as you are diagnosed (or currently still symptomatic), get the following items:

- A peaked hat and sunglasses for being outside
- Silicone ear plugs for social situations and sleeping
- Noise-cancelling headphones for home life if you have others in the house
- Eye mask for sleep and desensitisation

- A weighted blanket (if you like the sensation) to calm anxiety
- Sticky notes (for reminders)
- Journal to track symptoms
- Migraine glasses (with a rose-tinted lens may help)

THE DOWNWARD SPIRAL

By the time I got home, I couldn't remember anything the concussion physio had said, apart from the fact I was to be *unemployed, unable to drive and had to give up all my vices.* I called my husband, matter-of-factly delivering the news: 'I've been put off work with concussion. Can you pick up some sleeping pills from the doctor?'

He sounded worried. 'Oh babes, are you OK? Yes, of course, is the script there?'

I was stone cold emotionally and discharged a moment to flick the serpent's tongue in his direction. 'Yep, great. That's why I have a black eye, I'm having headaches and it feels like I've had a stroke on one side of my face.'

My acid tone was stopped short by him saying 'Okay, well I'll get the kids and take care of dinner, and you get into bed and rest.'

The line went dead.

I stood staring at the phone like an anthropologist discovering a new species of mammal. Then terror entered my brain like a crack of lightening as I realised what being 'off work' meant. *Hold on, I can't just stop! I've got work to do!* I'd been given a diagnosis which explained *everything and nothing* at the same time.

I contacted work and told them I would take the next three days to hand over the projects. 'It's concussion. I've been put off work for who knows how long. Can you . . .' Email after email, phone call after phone call – everyone just seemed to respond as if I'd told them I had a cold sore. 'Oh, that's no good, you'll be fine, just take a rest.'

Crawling into bed, I Googled 'Mild traumatic brain injury' until my eyes started to pulse on the screen.

The next day as I stopped drinking the caffeine and alcohol, my world quickly crumbled into chaos. Without the dopamine hit to wire my neurons together, my brain said, *'Screw this, we're taking the year off* and left the cerebral hotel to holiday somewhere warmer.

My brain ground alarmingly to a snail's pace. I still felt the pressure to get the work handed over, but it was like knitting a sweater without needles. My speech slowed to a slur and as I walked down our stairs my body was completely off balance; I held the handrail with a death grip. When standing, I needed a chair to remain upright. I had to completely come off the computer and phone, because every screen was like a firing line of brain bullets. I was scared. I didn't know what was happening to me, and it all felt as if it was *out of my control.*

Feeling fragile and unsupported by my husband, I contacted a friend who was willing to move in with our family to support my recovery and manage the children in my current state. She offered to move in that weekend to help run the home.

But as the week progressed it felt like a great 'unravelling'. My smooth motor function dulled, and my sensitivity heightened. Noise, light and even talking felt like an ultra-marathon. I was taking the prescribed sleeping pills and still couldn't sleep. My brain racing like I was at a concert, as I lay wide-eyed on the couch eating toast.

Each sunrise brought intense nausea (like the worst pregnancy), and everything irritated me: the kids laughing, the cutlery being put away, the husband chewing his breakfast, the dog licking his paws. *Oh my god, somebody shoot me.*

Our normal morning routine became a torture chamber, and emotionally I was ready to explode. Then as the family finally left for school and work, I was left in a haze of silence. I would sit crying on the couch with a large hooded cloak over my eyes, listening to the sound of the clock ticking.

On the worst day of that week, I decided to drive to a local bush track for a walk. My ears felt as if I was in a plane at high altitude, and I ended up sitting at the base of a tree for hours, not knowing how I got there, where I was or why. Somehow I had left my body and all that was left was a lumpy human shell. The only reason I returned home was that my husband called to see where I was.

The extremes of emotion were intense. The white rage of the external factors (noise, light, the pain) and then a hollow sadness when my world was quiet. I didn't understand on any level what was happening to me. All I understood was that I did not want anyone around me, yet when I was alone I felt like a dark empty blanket of nothing.

Support

Once you are diagnosed it is vital to have a support team. Your brain is compromised, and you need people to know what is going on.

Your team need to know you will be experiencing:

- Fatigue

- A reduced ability to do normal tasks
- Irritability or sadness when overwhelmed
- Headaches when exposed to too much noise or light
- A need to avoid lots of people
- A poor memory
- Mood swings
- A lack of social skills

It is also beneficial for your support team to know what activities you may need help with, for example:

- Being driven to appointments or driving to engagements
- Being an advocate in appointments
- Increasing help around the home
- Cooking meals and cleaning

Emotional support

At the beginning of this journey, whoever is in your life will be going through the journey with you. It is very normal when you have a head injury to experience:

- Anger
- Grief (for the person you were)
- Sadness
- Frustration
- Wanting to be alone

Many of these feelings arise when you need a 'brain break' and the greatest tool is to tell them you need a time out before you explode these emotions onto them. For a brain injury, taking time out can be the greatest healer. This can be a walk (or some other physical exercise if you can), meditation or a brief power nap without stimulation to recharge the brain battery.

Screen time

Get off all screens immediately in the early part of your recovery – your phone, the TV, the computer. Anything that provides external input into your brain. You need this time to rehab and rest. As reading may be difficult, find an alternative activity to fill your day like colouring in or gardening. If you need to use screens, switch everything to *'night mode'* which reduces blue light. A screen filter or tinted glasses can also help.

Caffeine

There are conflicting studies, but caffeine is known to be inflammatory for the brain. It also stimulates your nervous system, which is already overstimulated. You are likely to have a few days of withdrawal if you are a regular coffee drinker, as your body remembers to make your own energy again. Take all forms of caffeine out of your diet immediately to allow your brain to heal:

- Coffee
- Black tea
- Sodas with caffeine

Switch this out to herbal teas or green tea (has caffeine but also l-theanine which calms the brain).

Alcohol

Alcohol interferes with the brain's communication pathways and can affect the way the brain looks and works. Alcohol makes it harder for the brain areas controlling balance, memory, speech, and judgment to do their jobs, resulting in a higher likelihood of injuries and other negative outcomes. It is a toxin and a poison to your brain. Take all forms of alcohol out of your diet immediately.

Understand your triggers

Knowing your personal triggers is very important (see traffic light chart in the appendix). The traffic light is a tool to communicate with your loved ones which 'colour' you are currently. If you are green, your symptoms are low, orange they are starting to manifest (pain, fatigue, anger) and red is the danger zone. When you know what makes you symptomatic, you can explain to others that if you are around these things, you will need to take a brain break before and after. For example:

You need to travel in the car to a family function, yet driving is a 'red trigger' currently. Take a brain break when you arrive at the family function with noise-cancelling headphones for 15 minutes.

When you get to ORANGE, you need to take a brain break. Some triggers can include:

- Social situations
- Loud music or television
- Travelling in the car as a passenger
- Being outside
- Driving
- Cooking (if smells make you nauseous)
- Talking or listening for too long
- Loud voices

Chapter 4

The suicide attempt

'We are such stuff as dreams are made on; and our little life is rounded with a sleep.' The Tempest, William Shakespeare

Despite taking the sleeping pills regularly, they hadn't worked, and after a week of no sleep I was like burnt toast. A heavy cloud settled over my brain, and *everything* was annoying me.

It was the night before my friend was moving in with us and my husband saw a 'window' of opportunity. As we lay in bed, he nervously said 'Hey, umm – Jeremy is going fishing in the morning, and I, aaah – wondered if I can go with him?'

I looked at him coldly. Sleep deprived and emotionally drained, I asked 'What time?' He smiled, excited for some freedom from his routine of work and extra parenting. 'Oh early, I'll probably leave here at 5.00am. You'll still be in bed with the kids. I'll go fishing and then I'll pick up the duck-shooting license in town and be home at lunch time. Oh, and then I'm going out with Adam duck shooting after that. You remember that, aye?'

Fishing, *then* duck shooting? An *all-day* adventure? I didn't remember this nor any conversations we'd had for weeks. I blew out a sigh, then relented. 'Sure, that sounds fine. So I'll have the kids on my own all day?' I was still unsure of my ability to parent alone as I couldn't even walk without feeling I was going to collapse.

He replied cheerily, 'Well, your friend's arriving tomorrow, isn't she?' My eyes darted side to side; I had completely forgotten she was coming. *Oh yes, my friend, another lifeline.* 'Yep, whatever, go and do what you need to.'

Excitedly he packed for the next day, his one excursion of hunting and gathering. As he rustled in the drawers, I rolled over in bed and silently wept with my brain pounding in a million different ways.

That night despite the prescribed pills, the warm blankets and the deep breathing of my husband next to me, I lay awake until the early hours listening to the fluid rushing in my head. I must have had a brief nap before dawn though because when I woke my husband was gone. And boy was I angry! The feeling that he had '*left*' me alone turned from abandonment into rage.

The children rushed in for their morning cuddle, and I yelled at them to leave me in peace. The TV was quickly switched on as I stumbled down the stairs to play parent. Noise splintered into my brain. Making breakfast, doing the housework and trying to be a mother – while my eyes felt as if they would fall out of my skull at any moment.

Each time a TV character giggled with glee, I felt knives stabbing. I whispered to the kids, 'Can you turn that TV down, guys?' 'But Muuum, it's really low already.'

I walked out of the room and sat on the stairs with my head in my hands.

In just a few days my life had unravelled. I realised I wasn't important to my job or my husband, and as long as there was food and a screen I wasn't important to my children. The more I Googled mild TBI with my eyes burning at the phone, I felt as if I wasn't 'mild' at all. I'd had enough.

When my husband arrived home at 12.30pm, I was fried and angry. I didn't care that the children were right there; having no filter on my emotion, I was out for blood.

As he walked in the door after a wonderful morning of fly-fishing, I started screaming. 'I need to sleep!' He blinked, as if he'd walked into a sandstorm. 'But I'm meeting Adam at 1.00pm to go duck shooting.'

My blind rage erupted onto him. 'Screw you! I'm injured and all you care about is hunting. You leave me with the kids and go off hunting. Screw you! Screw you! *Screw you!'*

I was out of control. I flew towards him, anger pouring out of me like a death ray – I felt as ifr I could kill him. He held me off and started yelling back. 'I don't have any time to do what I want to do.'

The children ran to keep us apart and cried, 'Stop it, Mama! Stop yelling at Daddy!' Then I fell to the floor in a wailing heap. Their small faces blurred amidst my tears. Feeling they were all against me now, I got up in a frenzy and shrieked 'Screw you all!', running upstairs to lock myself in the spare room.

On the other side of the barrier there was silence. My heart beat loudly inside my head.

Then light footsteps and a gentle knock. 'Muuum! Muuum! Please come out.'

Heavier footsteps, then my husband was outside the door as well. 'Come on guys, come and watch TV, Mum's not feeling well.' Their tiny footsteps drifted away. It felt like the story of my life to come, a feeling that everyone was just moving away from me.

I ripped open the door and my husband was still standing there. I bared my teeth like a rabid dog and spat. 'Screw you, I've had no sleep and all you can think about is yourself and your stupid hunting.' He was still overtly calm, which angered me even further. 'Look,' he said. 'I'll take the kids with me, and you can sleep. Get some rest, babes. You'll feel better if you get some sleep.'

I screamed at him at the top of my lungs till my voice bled with pain. Screamed till the demons raced at his head and tore the flesh off his skull. *'Screeew you!'*

I ran into the storage cupboard under the roof and sat in complete darkness sobbing. Tears ran hot down my cheeks like melted wax, my head pounding like a potato on high in the microwave. 'Screw you,' I whispered. 'Screw you all.'

Outside, I heard the doors of the truck shut. My little girl's voice: 'Is Mama okay, Dad?' My husband replied, 'She's okay, babes, she just needs some sleep.'

I sat there rocking in the grip of insanity. In my mind I'd been left alone all week to look after the children and felt I didn't matter to my husband or anyone else. I was toxic and out of control.

Then a thought occurred to me – *'I just need sleep'*. Yes, I absolutely did. I would be better if I could *just sleep*. So as the truck rolled out of the driveway, I ran to the bedroom and popped two sleeping pills. Yet after a few minutes, nothing happened. So I ate two more, then two more, and two more – just to be *sure* I could sleep.

I remember vaguely walking down the stairs to get my *entire* drug supply of antidepressants, migraine pills, antihistamines and ADHD pills and putting them all in a large bag to take to bed. With a bottle of water, one by one with no memory of how many I swallowed, I gave myself the gift of sleep. Goodnight. Lights out.

Sleep

Sleep is a basic biological need for all mammals on the planet. If a person is deprived of sleep for longer than 24 hours, mental and physical problems begin to develop. Researchers believe that during sleep we remove waste products from the brain. For concussion it is the one thing that will refuel the tank effectively.

The first signs of sleep deprivation are fatigue, irritability and brain fog. Then we are unable to concentrate, speak clearly, our judgement wanes, body temperature lowers, and our appetite increases.

If the insomnia continues, disorientation, social withdrawal, depression and even hallucinations can start to occur.

It is imperative to find a way to sleep early on. If you cannot reach full sleep, then practising meditation and deep breathing can support in many ways. For the people around you, monitoring your sleep habits will be a key rehabilitation tool.

If you are finding it hard to sleep:
- Do not go anywhere near a device for three hours prior to bed.
- Use noise-cancelling headphones to listen to binaural beats, brown or white noise or a guided meditation.
- Use silicone ear plugs in bed.
- Have blackout curtains or use an eye mask.
- Use lavender essential oil on your pillow.
- A warm shower or bath before bed with lavender.
- Consider taking magnesium glycinate to help with relaxation before bed.
- Practice deep belly breathing (in for a count of three and out for a count of seven) to calm your nervous system.

- Ensure you are not hungry before bed. Having a snack of protein can support blood sugar drops which may wake you up.
- Ensure your room is not too warm.
- Sleep with socks on – when our feet get cold this can cause a drop in body temperature that can lead to frequent waking in some people.

Rest

Just like a broken bone, your brain needs rest to heal. It is crucial to know how much you can do before you feel fatigued and plan your rests during the day. The danger with concussion is that you overcook your chicken, and then pay for it later. So when you start feeling symptomatic, aim to have mini brain breaks. It can be helpful to set a series of alarms so that you know when it is time to stop and let your brain rest.

Don't let yourself get to the point of fatigue before you rest as this will cause emotional symptoms to raise their head.

You may structure your day so that every chunk of activity has a chunk of rest *(see resource section)*.

🧠 *Binaural beats and EMDR*

The pain was intense and when I couldn't sleep, I found binaural beats to be extremely helpful for pain and fatigue. Not only was there brain pain, but there was also leg pain, neck pain and shoulder pain. Pain everywhere.

Six months after the initial injury, I went to the library and found a book called *Change Your Brain, Change Your Pain* by Mark Grant MA, who writes that 'long term pain is in the brain'. When I read that, I was angry! Because I could feel the pain in my body. But the book demonstrated a pathway along with meditations that could ease pain in the brain.

During the first months of the injury, the pain may be located at the site of impact. Yet ongoing pain is due to the electrical signals in the brain, which may be helped by exercises to rewire pathways.

I was willing to try anything, so every night I would listen to the Mark Grant EMDR meditations. Suddenly I was sleeping better, and I felt as if I had more control over the pain in my body. See resources at the back of the book (EMDR specialist Mark Grant MA).

Binaural beat therapy is an emerging form of sound wave therapy. It makes use of the fact that the right and left ear each receive a slightly different frequency tone, yet the brain perceives these as a single tone. I also found these very calming to use for 'brain bathing'.

TO THE EMERGENCY DEPARTMENT

Hours later I floated down the stairs to find my friend in the kitchen unpacking. She later told me that I had dumped at least 20 empty pill trays on the kitchen table in a plastic bag and I'd said, 'I think I've overdosed – call an ambulance.'

It was dark when the ambulance arrived. A blur of a memory – two people in uniforms ferrying me onto the sterile gurney, fluorescent lights, the equipment shining brightly. As I sat in the vehicle, my friend sitting beside me, I heard my family pull into the driveway. Murmurs from outside, I could hear my kids yelling 'Mum! Mum! – is Mum okay?' The medic spoke in whispers to my husband then to my friend.

My friend leant toward me gently, 'Simon wants to come – I can get out.' Slurring my words, I babbled 'He doesn't care about me, leave him with the kids.'

I closed my eyes, and for the first time in weeks I disappeared into a dark rest.

When I awoke in the hospital I was attached to several beeping machines. The doctor shone light into my pupils. I can remember saying 'Do you know you have three eyes?' Then sleep swallowed me again.

As I travelled in and out of consciousness, the nurses were in and out checking the machines, the clinical heartbeat like a constant tap dripping. My friend held my hand close by. 'You okay?' she'd ask, and then my eyes would close again.

My attachment to the real world was wavering, and I felt pulled deeper into the dream time that never ended, with a storyline I knew well.

I was seeing my life in 'backwards play'. I remember this moment so vividly, as though stored in a memory box inside the brain: moving into our new home, my marriage, the births of my children, memories of acting and drama school, the awkward teenage years. Flashbacks of being a child at the beach with my mum and dad, right down to standing in my wooden cot at six months of age, screaming for someone to come in. But as the white wooden door with the plastic 70s turn handle opened, suddenly, my eyes flicked open.

I was back in the hospital bed and could suddenly 'see' again. *Months later a therapist told me that I was very close to death as the 'backwards show' is often a sign we are on the way out of earth school.*

'Why did you do it?' my friend asked, with her beautiful green eyes staring at me. I didn't understand. She continued, 'Why'd you take all those pills?' *Oh, now I remembered where I was.* 'I was tired,' I whispered. She squeezed my hand. 'Why didn't you call me, I could have come out earlier.' Struggling to keep my eyes open, 'I was tired, and taking the pills seemed like a good thing to do.' She laughed. 'That's a lot of pills, bro.' I smiled. 'They weren't working very well, so I kept going.'

By midnight (or whatever time it was) I was wired. We were laughing, telling jokes and I'd hijacked the nurses' rubber gloves to blow up into hand balloons.

The night nurse poked her head through the curtains, looking confused. 'You had sleeping pills, aye?' I laughed, obviously without any realisation of the severity of what I had done. 'Yep, a truck load.' The nurse shook her head, 'I've never seen anything like it, what you took would have bowled a horse over.'

Without any sense of a filter, I burst out laughing. My friend laughed as well, with tears in her eyes. Nothing was funny about the situation at all, but just in that moment I felt happy – the happiest I'd been in weeks. Suddenly my brain was clear, no headache (probably due to the excess of migraine pills). I could talk without slurring my words, and I felt that the light which had been ripped out was back on again. I could even remember giving my friend my shoes in a will I had written on the back of scrap paper (which she politely declined). 'They wouldn't fit you,' I joked, 'they're way too big for your short ass.' I laughed manically, as the beeping of the machines lulled me back into the dreamtime.

It was morning when I woke, and my friend was still there. The nurse poked her head in. 'You okay?' I felt amazing. 'Yep, sweet as. Can I go?' The nurse looked back towards the triage team. 'Just wait for the doctor to sign you off, and then you can go. I think the mental health team want to meet with you today, just to check in, okay?'

The entire night had felt like a dream and all I could see was that my symptoms were '*gone*'! The pain, the emotional issues, all felt wiped clean. My friend gathered up her things. 'Look, Simon is coming to pick you up, so I'll go. Will you be okay?' I smiled, replying as though she had just made dinner, 'Yep. Thank you for saving my life.'

She took a breath and lowered her voice. 'Seriously, I thought I was going to lose you there for a minute. You were so white, and your jaw was all sunken in, like those dead horses you see on TV.' She looked at me intensely. 'Don't ever do that again, okay?'

I didn't connect with the seriousness of what I had done and flippantly replied, 'All good – thank you.'

When my friend left and my husband arrived, I gave him a kiss and a hug as if we'd been out on a date and everything was normal. It was very strange, almost as though *my brain had erased the previous night.* When I saw the mental health team it was like the evening was a bad dream and they were talking about an event that I literally had no emotional connection to.

We walked across the hospital carpark to the mental health crisis team office. In the musty 1970s wallpapered therapist room I slumped down on a second-hand threadbare couch. The counsellor sat across from me in her floral dress holding a clipboard asking me with grave concern 'Why did you do it?'

I felt nothing. No emotions surfaced and I felt like I was talking about an accounting problem. Completely rational, I replied, 'I was tired and couldn't sleep and it seemed like a good idea to keep taking more pills.' I could vaguely remember my rage towards my husband for leaving me alone, but the intention behind the overdose was needing sleep, not wanting to die at all.

The therapist looked puzzled, made a few notes on the form and said, 'Well if you do need us, we are only a phone call away.' I offered to give her some natural health advice if she ever needed anything. The incident felt almost comical. The doctors made sure I was taking my antidepressant and ADHD medications regularly, but I was no longer allowed sleeping pills.

As we arrived home, my little girl clung to my legs. Looking up into my eyes with wide expectation, she asked, 'Why did the ambulance take you away, Mama?' I hugged her close. 'Mum's brain is a little bit damaged, babe; it's going to get better now.'

Suicidal ideation

Many individuals with a history of TBI never experience suicidal thoughts, yet research suggests that individuals with a TBI history may have increased risk of suicidal ideation. When I was 23, I was in a dark place of depression and intentionally tried to take my life, so I understand the feeling of not wanting to be on the planet.

What I know about feeling suicidal:

1. There is a feeling the world is better off without you
2. It feels like an escape from the hell inside your head
3. You may have lost purpose or identity
4. You may be physically unwell and want relief

What I want you to know as an individual:

1. You are loved by someone. Whether it's a family member, or your community, or a pet, something needs you here on the planet. The world is better with you in it.
2. You need help and someone to talk with to unpack these emotions.
3. Telling someone you are feeling this way will help you to feel better, or at least identify what you are thinking. It is likely you are in pain, or you are tired. Know that these symptoms will heal in time.
4. Do not go through this alone. There is light at the end of the tunnel.

What I want support people to know:

1. The attempt is not about you. It is a cry for help or an escape from their inner torment.
2. Watch for signs of going quiet, sending messages of 'Thank you' or giving away personal items.
3. For someone with concussion, in the early stages you must manage their medication and place it somewhere locked so that there is no unconscious action.
4. Know that lack of sleep is a form of torture and will cause your person to act irrationally. In the weeks following a bad concussion, make sure there is someone close by who can check in.

5. Speak to your person openly about 'suicide'. If you suspect they are withdrawing from you, ask them 'Are you thinking of taking your life?' If they say yes, ask 'Do you have a plan?' Although this conversation may seem confronting, you may save their life through being direct. You need to park discomfort and always enter open communication.

SETTING MY HAIR ON FIRE AND OTHER DUMB STUFF

After the suicide attempt, my husband took a week off work to look after me at home. The days were a blur as the drugs worked their way out of my system. I had been pushed up the 'urgency' list for the concussion team, however, and was due to have an assessment that week, along with a Zoom meeting with another concussion specialist to assess how severe the head knock was.

I was slowly becoming like a person with dementia. Small daily tasks that were once easy became major events that my brain could not cope with. I didn't remember simple conversations. Talking with my husband about the business was filled with 'I don't remember that', and I would act with complete surprise when he mentioned anything from the past. I'd walk from one room to another and completely forget why I was there; I burnt dinners, left hot taps running, and overflowed baths.

The height of the Alzheimer's came four days after my hospital discharge when my husband and I decided we needed to 'spring clean' the garage. Amongst the stored junk was a pack of tarot cards from my youth. Inside my mind I felt as though I was 'cleansing myself' of the evil spirits that had caused me to fall and bang my brain, so I decided to put the cards into the fireplace inside that was still smouldering from the previous night. The thick paper didn't even smoke, so I went to the shed and got turpentine and generously doused the pack. Nothing happened. 'Odd,' I thought, but determined to banish the metaphysical object, I got a business card, lit it, then threw it into the fireplace.

Suddenly a ball of light exploded out of the opening onto my face and hair. Turning to the mirror behind me, I saw a white fury of flames all over my head. Screaming, I ran outside patting the fire with my hands.

My head was smoking and my face hot as my husband ran from the garage. He wrapped me in his arms. 'Oh gosh, babes – what did you do?' I was shaking violently as he brushed his fingers gently through my hair, clumps coming away in his hands.

I felt small and frail inside his grip and so scared, so very scared. Something in my brain was wrong and I was out of control with no understanding of what was happening to me. I whimpered, 'it just seemed like a good idea.'

As I pulled the matted singed hair from my head and threw it onto the lawn, I started to sob. My husband pulled me close. 'Babes, it's okay. We'll get it sorted, we'll get it sorted.'

I smelt like cooked pork and when I looked in the same mirror where I'd witnessed my flaming hair, my eyelashes were down to little nubs and the eyebrows were gone. My skin had this impressive glow to it, though, the only half-cup-full moment of the day. Like a mutilated doll given a haircut by a toddler, I laughed 'I look like I've had a bad beauty treatment.'

Stay in the room and stay safe
During your concussion the brain is healing. Your capacity for taking in information is limited and too much stimulation will scramble the circuits. The best advice I had from one of my therapists was to 'stay in the room until the job is done'. Before the head injury I used to be able to multitask and flit from one activity to the next and return without worry. But during the rehabilitation I found my homing pigeon was more like an

ADHD squirrel. If I left a task, it was almost as though my brain had deleted the memory of where I was.

The brain's efficiency moves to 50 per cent when you start multitasking. Let your catchphrase be 'one thing at a time'. If you are making dinner, stay in the kitchen until it is done. Wherever you are, stay there until the task is completed. If you are cooking or running a shower and walk away, you may risk an accident. I found using post it notes very helpful for listing activities for the day and would leave these somewhere I could see them to remind me of what needed to be done.

Do not do anything alone that could risk your safety, like lighting fires, operating heavy equipment, climbing ladders or do-it-yourself projects in the first months following your concussion. If your prefrontal cortex (the rational brain controller) is damaged, you are more likely to engage in dangerous behaviour that could hurt you further. *Ensure that you have a support person with you; or, better yet, don't do it at all.*

Chapter 5

Rehabilitation

'You can't wring your hands and roll up your sleeves at the same time.' Patricia Schroeder

Two weeks after I set my head on fire, I had my first appointment with Vicki Gould (see resource section), an occupational therapist on the concussion team who was there to assess the severity of the brain injury. I still wasn't sleeping well and spent most of my days sitting on the couch with a large grey poncho covering my head eating toast. Without any screens to distract me, the hours dragged by, and I could cry at the drop of a hat. When Vicki arrived, I felt as if she was a character in another dream moment.

She asked me what I had been doing and my symptoms, and confirmed that these were all normal reactions to concussion. Vicki then tested my eyes with her pen and noticed that my 'midline' (where you perceive the centre of your body to be) was off and recommended that I get referred to a neuro optometrist to get assessed.

I laughed. 'So I'm not crazy then, I am actually on a lean?' She tested my balance – fail; my head movement – severe nausea; my speech, memory, symptoms – all failed. As a result, my ability to drive was firmly taken away until I was better.

She told me to plan and pace, which means that you do a little bit of activity and then rest. My homework was to do only five minutes of activity followed by five minutes of sitting in a dark space with zero stimulation. It was all part of healing the brain after concussion.

'You'll be assigned a case manager who you can call to arrange for taxis, as well as a cleaner if needed. Somebody will be able to take you to your appointments.' But then it hit me – for the first time in my life I was totally reliant on other people for my independence.

I whimpered, feeling totally useless, 'But how long until I'm better?'

'For some people it's weeks,' Vicki replied, 'and for some people months or years even. It's your brain, no one knows. I'll put these referrals through and see you later next week. Tell your husband he needs to help you. You need to stop everything you are doing and get better. If you don't plan and pace your day you will not get better. Quiet, more darkness, zero stimulation... okay?' Then she left.

I crawled into the cupboard of darkness under our stairs and cried – and at some point fell asleep.

Planning and pacing

With concussion, imagine you wake in the morning with a whole pie and each activity takes a slice. It is essential to plan and pace your day the night before to recharge the brain and avoid burnout.

In the beginning, you may do five minutes of activity, followed by five minutes rest. Or five minutes of activity, 10 minutes of rest. This will depend on where you start. As you heal, the level of activity may increase, but if you become symptomatic again, go back to the active/rest–active/rest formula.

Set a rest alarm on your phone (or get your support team to do this) until you are familiar with the habit. When you are planning your activity chunks make it small and achievable:

- Write down one thing you want to do that day (e.g. make your bed).

When you are pacing (brain bathing):

- Aim for zero stimulation during this time. If you have a dark cupboard, place a chair or beanbag inside and sit in there until you feel calm again. Using noise-cancelling headphones and an eye mask will help to refresh your brain.

As you heal you can add more things to your list for the day, but make sure that what you put on the list is important to you.

Don't add too many goals or anything that will overwhelm you in the beginning. You also will need to rest more the more you do, so be aware of the power of balance as you first begin to heal.

Create a coat hanger for your habits

The idea of this is extremely powerful. You find a habit that you currently do (like brushing your teeth) and you hang the new habit (e.g. belly breathing) onto it. This makes it easier for the brain to create an automatic trigger for the new behaviour. When you are beginning, everything will feel hard, but if you learn to 'coat hanger' basic tasks alongside your rehab, you will find that you start to automate habits and things get easier. It will depend on the level of your injury as to what you choose to coat hanger together and stack new habits on existing ones:

1. When I get out of bed – I make my bed

2. After breakfast I do my eye exercises for two minutes
3. After I do my eye exercises, I shower
4. After my eye exercises, I do eye palming

Another example may be (if you need to move more):

1. When I wake up, I will get dressed and put on my walking shoes
2. After my 10-minute walk I will eat breakfast
3. After breakfast I will do my rehab exercises for five minutes
4. After I do my rehab exercises, I will rest for five minutes

You can also use something to set an alarm if you want to create an audio queue for a behaviour. When planning and pacing, the alarm can remind you to spend time having a brain bath every hour to ensure your energy levels are topped up.

Chapter 6

Starting the work

"The greatest explorer on this earth never takes voyages as long as those of the man who descends to the depth of his heart." Julien Green

After Vicki's initial assessment I was fast tracked into the concussion team. This meant that I now had weekly appointments with her (occupational therapy) and a neuro physiotherapist and a psychologist who would visit my home.

Along with that, I was on the waitlist for various specialist assessments and had to navigate government departments to organise accident compensation and additional driving support.

Trying to speak to government organisations on the phone was like pulling teeth. Again and again having to repeat the same story, not remembering passwords for websites, or even understanding half of the actions that needed to be taken to tick the box on their system list. Many times I ended up in tears with a random customer service operator who was asking me to repeat my concussion story– when all I wanted was help. But eventually the tenacity paid off, and I qualified for taxi services to and from appointments and to collect the children from school, along with a weekly cleaner to help with domestic chores.

As I couldn't focus my eyes to read, and all screens were banned, my week went from vegetating on the couch to a throng of people coming in and out of the house with appointments scattered through the week. It was exhausting. Rehabilitation meant work that my brain resisted with all its might. Just talking to somebody else for longer than 10 minutes made me feel extremely tired. The normal hour-long appointments were like marathons. After each session, I would need to sleep for two hours.

Every new therapist came with a new set of exercises. When the neuro physiotherapist arrived, she assessed how my eyes were tracking and looked at balance and coordination. I was asked to walk a figure eight on the floor, which resembled a squashed pear. My body would not do what my brain wanted it to – I couldn't balance at all. I was given saccades to practice (which is just basic eye movement exercises to fire the brain), making me feel extremely nauseous.

I had a 'brock string' to try to correct my convergence issue. Letters taped on the wall to practise eye tracking. Neck stretches, compulsory daily exercise and my own regime of healthy eating. Amongst all the rehab, my pre-existing conditions were raised. Attention deficit disorder, anxiety and depression, the mental health battle that even though I was a naturopath wasn't solved without medication. Everything was worse mentally because of the head injury.

The psychologist would talk to me about the *comorbid* conditions of concussion, which I already 'had'. A head injury can make these pre-existing conditions worse (or create them in others). But the key was that 'if I healed my brain', these symptoms would also decrease.

We discussed my marriage, and each time my husband was used as a punching bag for the perceived lack of support. I was given more paperwork to read, and more exercises to do. The sessions made me feel as if I was more crazy than concussed, and afterwards I always felt sad and empty. Talking about how bad things were didn't seem to help at all . . .

After each session I would need to sleep for the rest of the day. Although the rehabilitation was meant to be helping, it seemed that I was digging holes in dry sand. Each step of progress was quickly followed by a caving in on itself.

As the weeks passed the specialists came to give me more exercises – more things I had to cut out, more things I had to do regarding eye movements, psychological tips, more stretches. They were all working toward the same goal (to get me better), yet I felt as if it was a mountain of work that didn't seem to produce results.

I was doing the planning and pacing, the eye exercises and meditating, yet the nausea of trying so hard to get better was burning both ends of the candle. I started to feel overwhelmed with the whole process and started to tell them what they wanted to hear.

I stopped everything and completely lied through my teeth when they arrived: 'Oh yes, it's totally improving. My knee? Oh yes, I'm doing those stretches every day and it is way better. My headaches? Oh yes, I'm doing the neck stretches, thank you, and they are really helping. Of course I am, yes, thank you so much, it is really working.'

I was able to pretend in those one-hour sessions that life was getting better. Yet, in truth, after they left I would sit back on the couch again feeling useless and disempowered. Staring into space, grieving the person I once was.

Some days I walked from room to room not even knowing why I was there. Some days I was so frustrated with the change that I wanted to rip my head off. Most days I would sob and sob when holding my family and felt frustrated that I wasn't even able to read my kids bedtime stories. I knew that everyone was just trying to help me, yet I felt helpless.

During the early stages of rehabilitation, Vicki the occupational therapist gave me the tools that felt like they were working to heal my brain. As I sat in the cupboard with my noise-cancelling earphones on, the silence was like a warm dark blanket that I cherished. The musty odour of the stored items and the soft wind that ran through the roof was the best part of my day. Some days I slept in the cupboard, some days I cried in the cupboard, some days I sat wide eyed and scared, as though this moment would never pass. Some days the anger overtook me, and some days I sat with nothing in my head at all.

Why me? Where have I gone? Why can't I just go back to how I was?

But I persevered with the rehabilitation. The neuro physio would try to touch my neck gently to ease some of the pain, but even the slightest touch felt like razor blades. I'd sit with the first young psychologist and discuss my triggers to try and settle my anger towards my husband. I said to her, 'If you turn up and I've bought 10 pigs and he's missing, you will know I've dealt with my triggers.' She blushed and smiled.

My mood was so up and down and dependent on how much 'pie' had been taken away from appointments during the day. Unfortunately my husband was still the punching bag for me, and I would sit outside with my friend at night (she was still living with us) bemoaning the fact that he was working when he should have been home with me.

Each day was so different, and I felt as if there was no stability in my symptoms or my mood. I was being given a lot of support to 'get better', yet my motivation to do the work was dependent on my energy. I knew I needed to trust the process. The hardest part was letting go of my former self. With a concussion a new vulnerability forms, and it is a scary road emotionally to just let go and trust.

Trusting the specialists

When you experience concussion, it can be like a glass bridge of healing. You cannot see whether each 'step' will help you. You need to have a certain amount of trust in those who are helping you. Often the healing happens in stages early in the rehabilitation; you may not feel like the specialists are helping, but it is important to keep on doing the work because eventually your brain will heal.

Comorbid conditions

If you have previously suffered from anxiety, depression, OCD or ADHD, you may find that your concussion makes these symptoms worse. It does not mean you are suddenly 'crazier'; your brain needs help.

Dr Amen has shown that specific foods and activities help the parts of the brain that are responsible for creating these symptoms (see resource section). Whatever your comorbid condition was prior to the concussion can be a clue to your healing pathway now:

ADHD: Your prefrontal cortex needs support

Depression: Your limbic system needs support

Anxiety: Your basal ganglia needs support

OCD: Your anterior cingulate needs support

The rehabilitation journey

Whether you have had a large brain issue or a small one, the following suggestions may help. Be aware that during the rehabilitation exercises YOU MAY feel sick. *With all the exercises, do them to a point of just feeling nauseous and then stop.* Consistency is better than quantity.

If you have had a bad day, do a little bit. The next day, do a tiny bit more.

You need three things before you begin:

1. A complete ownership of your health. Even though your medication and specialists are with you, they are only part of your toolbox to wellness. This is your journey and owning it 100 per cent will help you more quickly.
2. An acceptance of where you are right now, and knowing that each day will be different.
3. A sense of trust in the process. Some results may be immediate, others will take time.

The key to moving forward with your brain health after injury is to be gentle with yourself and celebrate the small wins.

For your brain it is like learning to walk again, and the information here is the full programme of my journey. Success did not happen overnight, but this gives you a pathway to follow as you get better. The rehab exercises that I found most beneficial were:

1. Eye saccades
2. Planning and pacing
3. Meditation
4. Balance exercises
5. Eye palming

Progress can be one step forward, two steps back

As your brain heals it is like a muscle getting stronger. Yet what can happen after the injury as we ADD more things into our day is that we can become symptomatic again. You may be feeling a lot better and then start working for a few hours. However, the headaches may start again. You may be working and add a new duty, then the headaches may return.

What I have found is that it is almost as if the brain is being stretched to accommodate the new information. Just like working out in the gym when the muscles tear to grow, the pain of progress is like this for a brain injury. Knowing that this is normal will help you to plan and pace as new activities or learning come into play.

Some things may have to drop off to let new things in and that's okay. You will eventually gather up your habits again.

Eye exercises

Saccades are eye movements that quickly shift the eye's focus between two fixed points. We use them when driving and when reading. Every eye movement that involves scanning our environment is a saccade. Healthy brains do this quickly. However, brain injuries and damaged neural pathways can lead to irregular eye movements.

The eye exercises that you are given to rehabilitate are very important. If you haven't been given eye exercises, here are some basic ones to get you started. I would recommend (if you are working with a physiotherapist) you get a specialist to guide you through these. With these exercises **only go the point of nausea** and then stop. Consistency is always more important than quantity. You may repeat these for one minute each, but please go at your own pace:

Move the eyes as directed (only one exercise at a time). Hold the stretch for 30 seconds; if you start to feel nauseous, stop and come back to it again later.

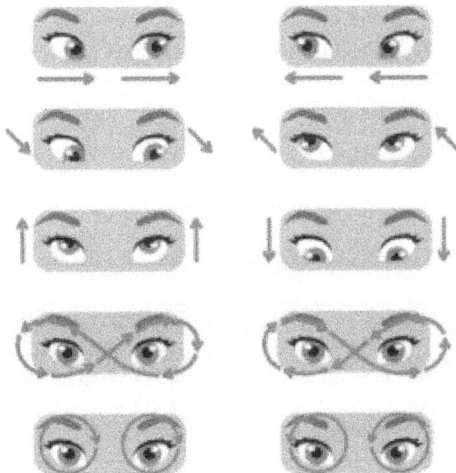

Additional eye exercises I used were:

- Tracing mazes on paper
- Eye stretches with eyes closed (holding a position like a muscle stretch)
- The Brock string (see Ryan O'Connor resources)

🧠 *Cross body exercises and balancing*

When you experience a concussion, you may find that one side of the body is weaker. Whatever side of your brain is hurting, you may find the opposite side of the body struggles to balance. For example, an injury on the right side of the brain may affect movement on the left. There are two hemispheres to the brain – the right and the left. In the middle is a bridge called the corpus callosum which transmits messages to either hemisphere. Whichever side is struggling is where your work is, but only ever go to your edge. If you use your symptom traffic light, i.e. if you get too red, you have gone too far.

Cross lateral movement creates connections from one side of the brain to the other, across that connecting highway, building the bridge between the two halves of the brain. It then creates the capacity for even more complex sensory processing, complex movement and complex thinking to happen. Basically it helps our brain to function better.

Incorporating cross body exercises and balance into your rehabilitation journey will start to fire up the bridge in your brain, leading to better cognition. Simple places to start:

1. Holding onto a support if you need to, balance on one leg
2. Brush your teeth with the opposite hand
3. Seated on a chair, place the opposite hand to the opposite knee and keep switching until you feel nauseous, then stop
4. Bear crawl
5. Hand clap game (any sort of alternate hand motion)
6. Holding ears and squat (Jim Kwik)
7. Ping Pong
8. Tossing a ball to a partner.
9. The cross crawl is a powerful brain stimulator that can also be performed on a chair.

THE CROSS CRAWL

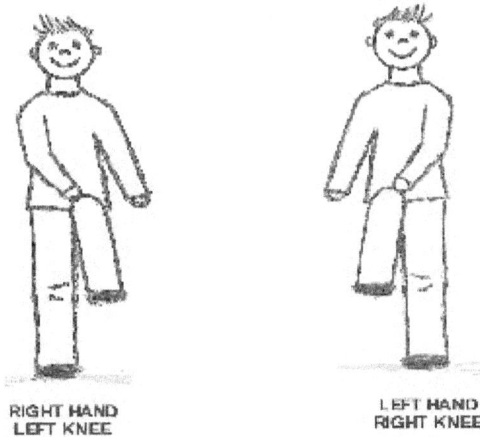

RIGHT HAND
LEFT KNEE

LEFT HAND
RIGHT KNEE

Eye palming

Palming originates from yoga and helps to relax the eye muscles. To palm, start by rubbing your hands together to warm them up. Close your eyes and place the palm of each hand over the corresponding cheekbone. Cup your hand over each eye and breathe deeply for five minutes. This can be a beautiful brain bath during the day.

THE NEW NORMAL

At home we started to settle into the new normal. In the mornings before the children went to school, I walked around with my noise-cancelling headphones and wore silicone earbuds anywhere there were humans. The wins for the day were:

1. Making my bed
2. Showering
3. Doing the rehab

My hat never left my head and if I was outside the sunglasses were on.

Days blurred into each other and each week the specialists would arrive and leave. I was doing the rehabilitation exercises daily and then would need to sleep to regenerate. I had come completely off social media, TV and reading, and I noticed how much even talking exhausted me. When my friend came home talking about her day, listening to her felt like worms eating into my brain matter. My kids enthusiastically bounded home after school inside and were immediately shut down to be *quiet* around the Mama.

One day my friend (who was still living with us) sent a video of a news article illustrating a building in burning flames somewhere else in the world and showing the people screaming. I cried for four hours after seeing the content.

When I mentioned this to Vicki the occupational therapist, she suggested I avoid watching the news, to protect my brain space. My emotional filter, the ability to disconnect from the outside world, was extremely thin. *I felt like a 'raw human' without any skin to protect me from 'words' or 'thoughts'.*

I avoided seeing anyone apart from my immediate circle because whenever I spoke with others it made me very tired. One friend came out to share some local gossip, but after she left I felt physically sick from the conversation.

The world continued without me, and I was in a bubble of healing. I was there, but not there, and it became accepted that whatever was happening with the family would *not* include me.

The children would ask 'Is Mum coming with us?' And my husband would reply, 'No, she has a sore brain.' Social gatherings, sports days, any type of outside event – I would be left alone in the house on weekends and my husband would take the kids. A blessing, though, because every time I was in a car, it triggered my concussion symptoms.

🧠 *Protect brain input*

Talking and listening may be hard right now. Your emotions will be riding high, and it is imperative to protect your brain while it's healing. It is crucial that the right ingredients are in place. Know what triggers you, and what makes you feel better. Avoid what hurts your brain, and harness what helps.

NEVER-ENDING WORK

The therapists came every week, and I would get another exercise, take something else out, until I was devoid of most things that I could use as a crutch. I didn't have much to look forward to: no social activities (by choice), no coffee, no chocolate, no alcohol, no cigarettes, no TV, no iPhone and no computer. But I still had carbs, and suddenly my salty-snack cravings were ON, making myself feel better by eating more potato chips, bread and crackers.

The team gave me handouts for my husband to read (which gathered dust). Multiple whiteboards were placed around the house to help me to plan and pace the day: post-it notes to remember where I was and what I was meant to be doing. I tried to engage my husband to plan the week with me – but he resisted. I would forget that his role of saving our business was a big job, as *my life box got smaller.*

Yet when you have no control, there is a tendency to try to create more. I started to obsess over the 'whiteboard'. I felt I needed to know exactly where my family was when they were out of the house. All I had to focus on was myself, there was no world outside my four walls. All my normal parenting duties were delegated. Between my husband, friend and parents, the cooking, cleaning and children were done. *I had no formal responsibilities.*

All I had to focus on was getting better, but I was still in pain and angry. I had no gratitude for what was being done for me, I just focussed on what I didn't have. I wanted my old life back and the rehab exercises were making me feel sick. Every day felt like a mountain of pushing uphill, and all I wanted was someone to *fix* me.

I was so tired of everyone telling me what I had to do to feel better. Where was the magic bullet? Despite all the painkillers, the migraine pills, the antidepressants, the nerve inhibitors and the ADHD medication, nothing felt as if it was working. I wanted control, but planning my rehabilitation and appointments were the only threads to humanity available.

Use a diary and whiteboard and calendar

In your diary (or get your support person to do this), write down the tasks that are important to do for you the next day. Schedule any specialist appointments as soon as they come in and make a habit of reviewing this first thing in the morning.

Use a calendar to make sure you schedule your appointments ahead. This is crucial for your support person to know what is happening as well.

What can be helpful is to write up what the whole family is doing (if you live with others) during the week, so you are aware of when people are in and out of the house.

Why planning is important as a household

Depending on the severity of your concussion, you may be in a place where you have little else to focus on. Your appointments may be the only real outside social interaction in your day, and it is very easy to 'lose' time outside these things. By planning the week, you can start to see that there are things to look forward to and start to regain control again. How this helped me:

1. Each night write down in your diary one thing that you would like to do the next day, e.g., weed the garden for 10 minutes.
2. Know what the family is doing, so you can actively understand what is happening in their world.
3. Focus on planning your rehab at a time when you can rest afterwards, e.g. 10 minutes of rehabilitation then 10 minutes in the cupboard.
4. Planning allows you to start to recreate structure in your day, when initially there may be none.
5. Routine helps us to feel like we are grounded and in control. Writing down the main things you need to accomplish that day: shower, eat, brush teeth and then ticking them off helps to build a sense of achievement.

SLOW BRAIN

I found that my brain was slow, and although I was in agony, some days when the family were out of the house I would sit outside for hours and watch the ants. I was completely reliant on my therapists as my lifeline to the external world. My appointments were the only structure I had created. It didn't matter if I didn't make the bed. It didn't matter if I showered. The longer I was out of the human rhythm, the less I had. It was very easy while not working to slip into 'I'll do it later', and then when the children came home with my husband in the evening, I would start to feel resentful that I hadn't got done what I wanted to do.

When I discussed this with my occupational therapist, she suggested creating a routine based on what I had to do. Starting small (amidst the stays in the cupboard) to create a structure in my day. Every evening, I would list what was important to me to get done for the next day. I started with small steps as she suggested.

1. Make my bed
2. Shower
3. Eat
4. Rest
5. Do the eye exercises
6. Rest
7. Exercise

By creating a rhythm in the day, I started to feel as if I was achieving more. I still wasn't doing all the rehabilitation suggestions (as my energy would deplete very quickly), but I was gently nudged by the specialists to start increasing my capacity.

On suggestion from the specialists that I had avoided was meditation. I used to do a lot of yoga in my youth but I was resisting adding another 'thing' to the pile of rehabilitation. Even though I was not meant to be on the 'screen', my curiosity peaked as to whether I could find a quick guided meditation to support my aching brain. I found a yogi online called Sadhguru, who teaches a technique incorporating meditation and humming.

This seemed like a more 'active relaxer' type of mindfulness that appealed to my ADHD brain. As I sat in the lounge with my noise-cancelling earphones on, the smooth voice lulled me into the *ultimate brain bath*. When I opened my eyes after 12 minutes, I felt as if I could 'see'.

Sadhguru mentioned something called 'the vagus nerve', which I had never covered in my years of naturopathic study. I was intrigued. Because the meditation didn't make me feel sick, it became a firm addition to the daily ablutions.

Creating structure

The brain thrives on certainty. For those of you going through a brain-healing journey, your certainty may have been ripped out. The normal pattern of getting up and going to work may be gone. The normal motivation to get things done may be gone. But to heal, it is extremely important to create a morning routine that will set you up for the day.

When you are setting up your morning routine, list on a piece of paper these things:

1. What will make me feel like I have accomplished something today? As simple as making your bed.
2. What will make me feel calmer today? It may be doing a 12-minute meditation.
3. What will make me feel energised today? It may be getting outside for some fresh air.
4. What will make me feel better today? Having a shower is a good place to start, and always ensuring you eat breakfast.

When you have your shortlist of things that will help, put them into a structure that you can sustain. If you have ADD/ADHD like me, you may want to make a massive list of 'to-dos', but *this won't work for concussion.* You are better to choose three to four items that you know you can achieve every day and build the foundation from there.

The vagus nerve and meditation

After a concussion, you move to a 'fight or flight' mode due to the sympathetic nervous system and the calming part of the nervous system (the parasympathetic) shutting down. This affects the vagus nerve (also known as the vagal nerves), the main nerves of your parasympathetic nervous system. This system controls specific body functions such as your digestion, heart rate and immune system. The vagal nerves carry signals between your brain, heart and digestive system.

The vagus nerve is important for you because it can help to regulate your nervous system and calm you down. Incorporating one of these suggestions in a daily practice can improve your mood and overall physical wellbeing. It is also unlikely to make you feel nauseous, which for brain bangers is a major bonus. Ways to stimulate the vagus nerve:

- Gargling with water for 60 seconds
- Singing or Humming (use in the cupboard) for two minutes
- Foot massage

- Cold water face immersion: immerse your forehead, eyes and at least two-thirds of both cheeks into cold water
- Laughter (funny jokes and stand-up comedy)
- Deep belly breathing
- Breathing through a straw for two minutes
- Combining meditation with the mantra 'Ahhh, Ohhhh, Ummm' as you are breathing deeply can help. Or you may like to use 'AHHHH, MEEEN'.

Chapter 7

Finding your why

'Effort and courage are not enough without purpose and direction.' John F. Kennedy

I still couldn't drive, but after six weeks of waiting I was off to see the neuro optometrist. A two-hour drive left me nauseous, with the windy back roads threatening to send my stomach through my mouth in several directions.

As I yelled at my husband to 'Slow down', my emotional bunny went on the boil. We fought again. This time with no escape from the metal cage, the blistering argument raked over losing the business', him 'not being around to help me', and ending with 'Well, maybe we should get a divorce.' As we arrived I was symptomatic, angry and full of blame.

As I sat in the waiting room for the neuro optometrist, sunglasses on indoors, my brain pounded. My husband sat across from me in the waiting room, head down, unsure of what was going to happen to our marriage.

'Mrs Jolly?' Brenton Clark poked his quirky head out of the office. Immediately I liked him. He reminded me of a mad scientist who was cooking up magic in his cave. He asked me about what had happened and explained what could be going on with my eyes in terms of my balance being completely knocked off kilter.

And then a pivotal moment occurred.

Before we began the rigorous testing, the neuro optometrist asked: 'Ms Jolly, what is the **ONE** thing from your old life that you want back?'

I took an inward breath. Not one person had asked me this in the months prior. Nobody had asked what was important to me in my rehabilitation. My 'why' – what was important to ME? It had all been about textbook exercises, taking stuff away, putting stuff in and mechanical rehabilitation that made me feel like a brain cabbage.

"Mrs Jolly, what is the ONE thing from your old life that you want back?"

I started weeping. It was so small, and yet at that time it was my everything.

'I want to be able to drive again so I can pick my kids up from school.'

As I sat on the leather chair in the quirky little office filled with books, skeletons and prisms, he adjusted his shirt and said firmly, 'Right, well the most important thing you need to be doing every day is your eye exercises – back and forth – just like you are at the intersection.'

I raised my eyebrows and laughed hysterically. My husband and the specialist gave each other the side eye from this outburst. 'What's funny?' Brenton asked.

Choking back laughter, I replied, 'I was told to do those weeks ago but haven't been doing them because they make me feel sick. I didn't connect with why I had to do them, so I stopped.'

I felt like an idiot. The one thing that could have helped me, I had stopped doing because I didn't understand *why* I had to do them. I had no *WHY*.

After two hours of intense testing my head was exploding, my nausea through the roof, but we had established that my brain had been kicked about an inch to the right. The OT Vicki was right in her initial observation that my vision was off, and the midline imbalanced. The good news, though, was that the problem now had a solution, and my new spectacles were going to be made and would be in my hands shortly.

'And once I have them, will I be able to drive again?' I asked meekly. The specialist smiled. 'Yes, Mrs Jolly, once you have your glasses you should be fine to pick your children up from school.'

My heart leaped. At last I had hope.

As we drove home, I was filled with a new sense of the future. Suddenly I saw how much my husband was doing for me. I reached over to take his hand. 'I'm so sorry for hurting you. I don't understand what's happening to me. You're the closest thing to me that I keep clawing. I love you . . .' He squeezed my hand tightly. 'We'll get there, babes. We'll get there.'

Leading the horse to water – drink it

Often we are given the tools to help our recovery, yet we don't implement. Sometimes, it can take many people giving us the same message until we finally 'drink' the water we need to heal. As with the specialists. They had all told me exactly what I needed to do in order to get better, but it wasn't until I had a clear 'why' that my brain understood the importance. If you can find your 'why' early on in recovery, your healing and ability to become disciplined with the advice you are being given will be fast tracked.

The neuro optometrist

A neuro optometrist deals with the diagnosis and treatment of vision-based problems caused by brain injuries. You may benefit from having your eyes tested as soon as possible. (See the resource section for more information regarding neuro optometry.)

Vision is our dominant sense. Dysfunction affects daily living:

- Driving
- Reading
- Hobbies
- Returning to work
- Balance
- Eye hand coordination

When talking with your neuro optometrist, ask them about coloured lenses to help with sensory issues as well. If you are having issues with the lights on indoors, often they will be able to prescribe a special filter to help the brain to calm down.

Feeling safe

The limbic system is the portion of the brain that deals with three key functions: emotions, memories and arousal (or stimulation). This system is composed of several parts, which are found above the brainstem and within the cerebrum. To calm down, we need to feel safe. This is why as humans we opt for routine over change, and this can manifest as all sorts of negative and positive habits. The key is to look for what makes you feel safe but also makes you healthy. Using these questions can help:

1. Who makes me feel safe and improves my healing?
2. Which activities feel safe and will improve my healing?
3. Which habits have I had in the past that will improve my healing and feel safe?

Hope is not a strategy – yet it can help you build one

Knowing that your brain can get better (from the proven work of Dr Amen) is a gift. It gives us all hope that life may be brighter than today. The quote 'Hope is not a strategy' is widely used, yet I feel the statement is incorrect. If we don't have hope, we have very little motivation to act. Hope combined with action is a game changer. Remember, even at your lowest point, if you have hope you have momentum to keep moving forward.

Know your why

Dr Amen (see the next chapter) has created a tool called 'The One-page miracle' which can be incredibly valuable to unpack your 'why'.

Take a quiet moment to reflect on these questions:

What do I want in my relationships with my:

Partner

Children

Extended family

Friends

What do I want for myself in these areas?

Physical

Emotional / Mental

Spiritual

Social (my relationships)

5 Reasons WHY I want to be healthy again?

1.

2.

3.

4.

5.

Chapter 8

Physical health

'Everyone has a doctor in him or her, we just have to help it in its work. The natural healing force within each one of us is the greatest force in getting well. Our food should be our medicine. Our medicine should be our food.' Hippocrates

Returning from the neuro optometrist with a newly found 'why', I had a sense of purpose and vigour. All the strategies from the specialists that I had been avoiding now seemed to connect and make sense. I wrote out a plan of things I should have been doing weeks ago and started to obsess on brain health. I climbed into my naturopathic studies to look at optimum nutrition, I was on a mission to get better quickly.

Studying what really helped the brain: exercise, nutrition, meditation, mindset – it was a fast inhale of information as the ADD hyperfocus clicked in. I discovered Dr Daniel Amen and his wife Tana Amen and read their book *The Brain Warrior's Way*, which brought together years of study into a brain health focus.

I ignored the 'no screen rule' and started to acquire my Google PhD in concussion. Dr Amen is quoted as saying 'you are not stuck with the brain you have' and I liked him a LOT. Suddenly I had hope. A tonne of it!

It was as if a switch had been flicked on because the couch surfer attitude was gone. Although I was still in a lot of pain, ultimately I was determined with a militant focus. *My brain would be better.*

Even though it hurt, and it would have been easier to not do it, I clenched my teeth to get moving again. I was finally listening to the specialist's advice after weeks of avoiding doing the work.

I had started earlier in the journey on a stationary bike on the advice of the physiotherapist, but after a few minutes I would feel sick. Yet the research told me that I needed high-intensity exercise, so I needed to push through the nausea and get the heart pumping. My new routine was that in the morning I got up and did 30 minutes of high-intensity exercise to oxygenate my brain. Hill climbs, bear crawls, intermittent training on the bike. Initially it made me nauseous and my knee ached, but then I noticed an improvement in my energy level for the day. Moving more meant I had more, and the cognitive wheels started to turn from just dedicating part of my day to moving the body.

I did the planning and pacing that Vicki recommended and changed back to a low carbohydrate diet (which had been my mainstay for years) to see what effect it would have on my brain. I removed all processed food and I learnt how the gut can be *leaky* after a head injury and how we must adjust and supplement to heal. I drilled over concussion research until my brain throbbed. What helps my brain? What harms MY brain?

I used a heart monitor to ensure that I was getting my heart rate up enough to have benefits. My friend and I would get up at 5.30 every morning and do hill climbs. I'd have a good protein breakfast, and by the time the kids were off to school in the morning I was back in the cupboard for my brain break.

I had found my why. Finally, after months of suffering, the light was shining at the end of a very long tunnel. Thank you, Brenton, and thank you to the team of specialists, I had found the key to my door.

Even things with my husband were better as I was no longer clawing at him or micromanaging his day by focussing on managing myself. Inch by inch I started to help with daily chores, dinners . . . and things were going well. I was *growing in the dirt* and the fixation with brain health was keeping my mind entertained, instead of thinking about the constant pain in my skull.

Move your body

In my past life I worked as a personal trainer, so I had a good idea of the benefits of exercise, yet that didn't extend at the time to brain health. I knew about dopamine, but moving was more for keeping the body fit – not for the brain. Depending on the severity of your original injury, exercise may not be available to you at this time. But the key factor we need to consider for brain health is that OXYGEN is the panacea for rejuvenating the brain. The reframe is: *'Movement is for my brain'*.

If you cannot physically exercise, then looking into hyperbaric oxygen therapy would be an alternative. The best way to start if you have any balance issues (like I did) is to begin by using a stationary exercise bike. This takes away any risk of falling and you can monitor your heart rate as you go.

In the beginning you may feel nauseous. Go to your edge, and the next day increase the time a little more. The goal is to elevate your heart rate. Depending on your physical capacity currently, choose an activity that works for you.

What I would suggest is remove all barriers. Time can often be a 'barrier', and so can travelling somewhere to exercise. My morning routine would involve getting up in my sleepwear and hopping straight onto the bike. I started with four two-minute exercise sessions during the day until I felt conditioned (not triggered).

If you can, physical exercise should be a daily non-negotiable, depending on the severity of your injuries. The key is to get your heart rate elevated for at least 20 minutes per day, pushing much needed oxygen into your brain.

This can be done in two 10-minute chunks or using the Tabata method for one 10-minute chunk.

The Tabata method can be a fantastic way to start. How it works:

- Warm up for two minutes
- Then for six minutes, work hard for 20 seconds, slower for 10 seconds. Repeating this cycle for six minutes.
- Warm down for two minutes

Nutrition – the largest piece of the puzzle

As a naturopath, I have tried many ways of eating over the years: vegetarian, vegan, keto, paleo and being a binge consumer of junk. In my 20s I was overweight and had fatty liver disease, my catalyst to study natural medicine. Yet never in all of my study did I consider or learn about the impact of food on the *brain. You'll notice this is a very LARGE chapter because you are what you eat,* and it will have a massive bearing on your healing. A simple rule of thumb with your nutrition is to ask two questions:

Is this hurting my brain?

Is this helping my brain?

Know there is a direct link between what you eat and how you feel.

As I studied the effects of good nutrition, then implemented what I learnt, my mental clarity went up. *The choices became about my brain, not my dress size.* I noticed patterns of symptoms being triggered when I ate badly. Certain foods (even healthy ones) would trigger migraines or brain fog, so I suggest you start to become mindful of what works for YOUR body.

Using a journal can be a fantastic tool (see food intolerances and triggers). Whatever level of concussion you have experienced, what you put into your body fuels it; more importantly, it fuels your brain. Your food can either lead you on a roller coaster of highs and lows or help your cognition. *Be mindful that when you are changing your nutrition, you need to notice what works for your body.*

In the beginning I wish I had known what impact a concussion has on the digestive system, because I would have avoided eating loaves of bread, sugar and potato chips. But there is a reason we do this because high carbohydrate foods increase tryptophan, and this *calms us down.* Yet in my experience we don't need the brain to run any slower.

When I started following concussion nutrition, I used previous knowledge of the glycaemic index and food intolerances to construct a plan. It was slow going, as I used trial and error to see what worked for my brain. To fast track your healing, I would recommend following *The Brain Warrior's Way* diet created by Dr Amen and his wife Tana Amen. The book shows different brain types and a full overview if you want to heal FAST. If you are a 'foodie' (as I wasn't during the concussion), Tana Amen has also written a cookbook, *The Brain Warrior's*

Way Cookbook, which shows you how to create brain-healthy meals.

Here is an overview of what I followed in the sections below.

Beware leaky gut

Up to three weeks after a traumatic brain injury your gut is leaky. This can cause nausea, bloating and stomach pain. You may find that you are craving sugar, which can be a major roadblock in getting your brain firing again.

In the early stages of your head injury for gut repair you may want to focus on the following:

- Clear soups or broths
- Full fat, no added sugar, Greek yoghurt (be careful if you have any sort of dairy intolerance)
- Gelatine (no sugar), which has amino acids to help heal the gut lining
- Mashed or well-cooked vegetables
- Low sugar protein powder
- Slow-cooked meat

These foods are soft on the gut and contain a lot of nutrients. If you think of transitioning a baby onto solid foods, these are the foods that will help, soft and easy to digest. Protein is packed with amino acids that help the neurons to dance happily in your brain.

Water

About 75-80 per cent of the brain is made up of water. Dehydration as small as 2 per cent can have a negative effect on brain functions. It can also exacerbate pain, which is a motivator to drink more if we know water will help. Dehydration and a loss of sodium and electrolytes can cause acute changes in memory and attention. *Each day make sure you are hitting at least eight glasses of pure water to help brain function.* If you don't like the taste of water, try the following:

- Add stevia-based flavour drops
- Drink it in the form of herbal teas
- Add sliced cucumber or mint
- Add lemon juice

Get a large water bottle to track your consumption. If you have low blood pressure, add some Himalayan salt and lemon juice, which creates a natural electrolyte drink.

A good recipe for an electrolyte drink is:

1-2 cups of water

Juice of ½ lemon

¼ tsp Himalayan salt

🧠 *Why you need breakfast*

One thing I didn't do well in the beginning was eat breakfast consistently, because I felt unwell. As soon as I understood the dynamics of blood sugars on brain health, I didn't miss breakfast again. When I skipped eating in the morning, I would be sniffing in the pantry for toast and butter before midday. Feeding your brain the right foods is key for recovery. Breakfast can be looked upon as 'breaking the fast', so whether you eat at 6.00am or 12pm the first meal sets your blood sugars for the day. Adding protein to this meal will help to stabilise your energy and mood. This may look like:

- An omelette with vegetables
- A protein powder smoothie with berries
- Greek full fat 'no added sugar' yoghurt with berries and nuts/seeds
- Poached eggs with vegetables on a very high fibre or low carbohydrate bread

Keep your blood sugars stable – avoid hypoglycaemia (low blood sugar)

Whether you are a brain banger or not, when we don't eat for a period our blood glucose drops. The condition is called *'hypoglycaemia'*, and the symptoms are very similar to the side effects of concussion:

Symptoms of Hypoglycaemia:

Headaches and migraine	Shakiness	Blurred vision
Brain fog	Anger/Irritability	Anxiety/Panic attacks
Insomnia or waking in the night	Restless legs	Mental confusion
Inability to concentrate	Palpitations	Depression
Flushing/Sweating	Racing thoughts	Lack of energy/motivation including depression

When we eat a lot of 'sugar' (including fruit and processed carbohydrates) our energy spikes and then drops out. When blood sugars are low, we experience a wide range of emotions from sad to angry. For anyone with a head injury, stabilising your blood sugars is key. *What you eat is directly impacting your brain health.* There are foods that will make you feel good and foods that won't, but understanding basic nutrition will allow you to make better choices. The Glycaemic Index (GI) is a standard tool to measure how quickly food becomes sugar in the bloodstream. By eating low GI, we can control the blood sugars and help the brain.

Foods that calm the blood sugars from spiking and help the brain:
<ul><li>Protein: meat, fish, eggs, seafood, legumes (beans, lentils, chickpeas, pea protein powder)</li><li>Fibre: All vegetables bar potatoes. Fruits such as berries, kiwifruit, citrus, apples and pears</li><li>Fats: nuts, seeds, olive oil, coconut oil, ghee</li><li>Grains: quinoa, brown rice, whole oats, legume pasta</li><li>Bitters: lemon/lime juice, vinegar</li><li>Herbs: cinnamon, sage, thyme, black pepper, oregano, sumac (all herbs have benefit, so add them to your meals)</li></ul>

Boot sugar

When blood sugars are too high or are fluctuating between low blood sugar and high blood sugar, this leads to activation of microglia (the brain's immune cells). This directly leads to an inflammatory cascade in the brain, or **neuroinflammation**. Sugar and processed carbohydrates (that quickly turn into sugar in the bloodstream) can contribute to inflammation in your brain. It is also VERY addictive, which causes you to overeat. When we know that the brain is searching for a little 'high' and this euphoria will leave you more symptomatic, it is a great motivator to *get off the sweet and focus on whole foods.*

Too much fruit in your diet (as these turn into fructose – another form of sugar) will also lead to overstimulation. If your system is deregulated, you may feel as if you don't want to eat. In this instance, utilise broths and a protein powder supplement to keep feeding your brain.

The best-case scenario is to aim for three main meals per day which consist of protein, fat and a good carbohydrate source. If you are hungry add in two low glycaemic index snacks. *Remember that if you are not feeding your brain properly, it will not function as well.*

Foods that spike blood sugars quickly	
Processed (if it's low fibre and high sugar beware)	Natural:
	Dates
Full sugar soda and juice	Dried fruit
Flavoured milks, low fat yoghurt	All sugars (except for xylitol, stevia)
Icecream, candy, chocolate bars (anything with added sugar)	Tropical fruit (pineapple, mango, etc)
White bread / crackers/ pasta/ flour	Honey
	More than two pieces of fruit per day
Jams and spreads, sauces like tomato/bbq/sweet chilli	

See the resource section on the Glycaemic Load to see what foods are 'green for go'.

Gluten – it may be worth eliminating

Gluten is a group of proteins found in wheat, barley and rye. We know that after a brain injury, up to three weeks later the gut permeability has increased. However, many people benefit from switching to a gluten-free diet. One of these proteins, gliadin, can cause adverse health effects in some people. The digestive system performs several very important functions in your body. In your digestive tract, your body breaks down food and absorbs nutrients into your bloodstream. If you have bowel issues, you may find a gluten-free diet beneficial.

🧠 *Food intolerances – track food is mood*

Keeping a food diary alongside your symptoms can be a fantastic way to notice how the food is working in your body. Note down what you eat, and then rate your concussion symptoms out of 10 (10 being the worst). The key is to notice the link between your nutrition and your symptoms. For example, using different breakfasts:

Food diary	Symptoms
Yoghurt and berries	Increased headaches 8/10
	Fatigued by 10.00am 9/10.
Eggs on high fibre bread	Headaches 6/10
	Fatigued by 12.00pm 6/10

🧠 *Foods that increase intercranial pressure*

The pressure inside your skull when you have a brain injury can be overwhelming. There are proven foods that increase this pressure which are important to be mindful of. Like food intolerances, you may want to rate your symptoms out of 10 using a food diary to see what certain foods do to your overall wellbeing.

Foods that increase intracranial pressure include:

- Sugar
- An **excess** of Vitamin A rich foods (sweet potato, pumpkin, carrot and beef liver are some)
- Aged meats and cheeses
- Alcohol
- Caffeine (this happens in some people)
- Excessive salt (normally through eating highly processed foods and drinking soft drinks)
- Pickled foods

Supplements

Everybody's 'body' is very different. What works for you may not work for another. I personally found these supplements to be very effective:

- Omega 3 Fish Oils – to help with inflammation and cognition
- L-Glutamine – to help with gut repair
- Magnesium Glycinate – to help with muscle relaxation and sleep
- Branch Chain Amino acids – improve brain function

- Ginkgo Biloba – helps brain function and cognition
- Melatonin – may help with sleep
- Phosphatidyl Serine – has shown to improve brain cell communication
- N-acetyl cysteine – has been proven to repair brain cells

There are many others that can help with mental health, but always check with your practitioner as they may affect the medication you are currently taking.

Add to your supermarket trolly as these nutritious foods are proven to help:

- Green tea – cognition
- Turmeric – inflammation
- Rosemary – memory
- Sage – brain health
- Raspberries – high antioxidant
- Sumac – high antioxidant
- Black pepper – stimulates the endocannabinoid system
- Ceylon cinnamon – helps to regulate blood sugars
- Thyme – cognition

Chapter 9

Mindset

'Love is patient, love is kind.' Corinthians

When you start feeling better, the risk is doing more than your brain can cope with. I was extremely fixated on my physical health and my mood started to go downhill. All I wanted to do was to work on healing my brain, rather than any other daily task. I started to lose patience with anyone who was disrupting my newfound self-improvement focus. I was doing the work, but the work was too much, and my brain started to struggle again.

My parents would visit on tenterhooks, not knowing what mood I was going to be in. My kids would cuddle up beside me, not knowing when I was going to lose my temper. Friends reached out trying to understand and offer me empathy, but no one knew the personal hell that was happening inside my head. I wanted to get better, but I wasn't there yet. I looked healthier on the outside, and I was doing more in my day, yet the bunny was on a slow boil to destruction.

After six weeks of following my military lifestyle, it was my nephew's birthday party. I still wasn't driving (as my glasses hadn't arrived) but I wanted to attend the event. The normal routine was that my energy would bottom out after a few hours of being awake, so after my 'sleep' in the storage cupboard we went to celebrate as a family. As we pulled up the driveway, there were seven other parked cars and immediately my heart started pounding. I had not been around that many humans since my hospital stay – and humans I didn't know!

As I got out of the car clutching my nephew's gift, the laughter coming from within was extremely loud. My anxiety climbed. I kissed my in-laws, put the present on the table, and found a quiet spot outside to blend into the background.

The reverberation of the children playing on the trampoline ate through every nerve in my body. I must have looked relatively normal, because another mother came up to me extending her hand, 'Hello, I'm Sam, who are you?' I smiled meekly and told her I was the mother of 'those two' (pointing to mine). She asked with the most beautiful smile 'What do you do?'

I felt my brain freeze and shrink, my palms hot, clammy and cold all at the same time. I blinked. My breathing was short and fast like a trapped animal. Head pounding, light glaring into my eyeballs like death rays, I had nothing – literally nothing. No answer, no social grace, nothing. My eyes filled up with tears and I said to her, 'I'm sorry . . . I've had a brain injury, and this is too much for me. I've got to go.' I quickly found my husband and asked him to drive me home.

Lasting just 10 minutes at the birthday party, I went home to the cupboard and cried, feeling like I would never be normal again. My diet was better, my exercising was improving, I was doing the rehab exercises and seeing the specialists weekly, but emotionally I felt fractured.

Go to your ledge but watch for symptoms

If I could go back in time and speak to my 'concussion self', I would tell her to watch for symptoms. Know that every time you add in something new, you can become symptomatic again. Even though what you may be doing is helpful, the key is to go to your ledge (until you notice triggering) and then rest. The process of rehabilitation is like teaching a child to walk again. There are going to be stumbles and moments where you want to quit altogether, because every day can feel hard. On those days you need more rest; take a brain break and acknowledge how far you have come.

Social engagements

When you are first starting to do 'human' again, please know that it is normal to struggle. Your brain is working differently; it may be slower. Noise and conversation can really tire you out. Even if you are feeling very well, find out about the situation before you go. Things that may help:

1. Be honest with people about your experience
2. Set a time limit on social interaction
3. Wear clear silicone ear buds to help with noise
4. Wear a peaked cap and sunglasses to reduce triggers
5. Make sure you are well rested prior to attending
6. Take a 'safe' person with you and let them know if you are feeling triggered

Journal

Writing, or using a voice recorder, can be a beautiful way to unpack what emotions you are feeling. Getting into a daily habit (before bed or first thing in the morning) can help to offload any negative thoughts.

Because it is scientifically proven that gratitude is beneficial for the brain, it will help you to start to journal three things you are grateful for in the day. Byron Katie created a series of questions to help you to navigate negative thoughts. When you have a negative recurring thought, you can journal using these questions:

Thought may be: 'I'm never going to feel better.'

1. **Is it true?** *(that I will never feel better again).* Your answer may feel like yes.
2. **Do I <u>absolutely know without a doubt</u> that it's true?** Your answer this time is likely to be no because you don't know it with 100 per cent certainty.
3. **How do I feel when I think this thought?** Pretty crappy, right?
4. **How would I feel if I didn't think this thought?** Better, I'm sure.
5. **What is the opposite of this thought?** Look for a possible answer. It may be: every day in every way I'm getting better and better.
6. **What evidence do I have that this new thought could be true?** Look back to your lowest point in your brain injury journey. Are you still as bad as you were? Or have you made progress but you're not seeing it?

THE BRAIN GLASSES

The day my new 'brain' glasses arrived in the mail was the biggest gift of my life. As the seasons shifted from autumn to spring, the murky grey day was illuminated with the neat little package. As I put on the amber-tinted lenses, my brain sighed, I kid you not. The world was suddenly on a tilt to the left – immediately my mind relaxed.

Oh, the excitement, the happiness. I really felt as though this was it. I was back into it again, and I could drive! Superwoman was back in full throttle.

The very next day, after months of doing nothing, I decided that I would exercise, do my rehab, drive into town and back, do the shopping, pick the kids up from school AND do dinner.

My husband suggested that he could pick up the kids and for me to do the shopping, just to ease into it. He was doubting my superwoman abilities, so I quipped 'Okay fine, if you don't trust me, you get the kids' and I drove into town.

Yet as I sat at the intersections again for way too long, cars mounted up beeping behind me. I could not navigate a right-hand turn as the oncoming traffic looked as if it was travelling faster than my ability to find a gap.

I pulled into the carpark at the supermarket (in a very crooked manner) and got my trolley. Word for the wise who know nothing of brain injury – the supermarket is like hell on earth for someone with sensory issues. Too many colours, too much stuff, too many humans and way too many fluorescent lights. *Bad move Mrs Jolly – bad move.* Immediately my anxiety climbed into overdrive.

I had a written list and underneath my baseball cap and amber-tinted prism lenses, I was tenuously holding sanity together. My grip on the trolley was moist and the flutter of my heart synced in with the humming of meat refrigerators. My brain screamed 'Get me OUT of here now!'

I sped round the aisles. The normal foods I bought had moved position in the supermarket. The brain started to boil the bunny. Inside my head a conversation began screaming:

'Have prices gone up? How can anyone afford this food and especially healthy food when these prices are what they are? Can that person go any slower? Are you serious? Get the f*** out of the aisle! You're talking now – in the aisle. Can't you see I'm going to explode? Move – I need to get some tuna!'

In that moment in the supermarket, with a hundred other humans present, I was going to lose my shit. The emotion whirled within my brain like a small dinghy in a storm. I opted for defeat with only half the list covered, my eyes filling with tears as I arrived at the checkout. A young girl served me politely, asking 'How's your day?' I kept my head down and managed a normal response 'Good thanks, and you?' She smiled, 'Good . . . not too busy for a Monday.' I wiped away a sneaky tear that had managed to slide down my cheek.

'Oh, that's good,' the credit card burning a hole in my palm. 'Would you like your receipt?' the young melodic voice enquired. 'No, thank you.' I removed all eye contact to avoid any further conversation.

As I packed the car, shaking violently, suddenly I heard a voice behind me. 'Katie!' It was someone I knew. Oh God, please no.

'Katie! How are you?' A friend I hadn't seen since lockdown was enthusiastically running over for a cuddle. I took a step back and she froze.

Her brown eyes darted side to side, as she asked again 'How are you?' She tried to keep up her enthusiasm, but she knew something was off. All I could manage was "Ah, I'm okay; had a head injury in lockdown.'

Then moments of uncomfortable silence as she waited for me to continue. Becoming quiet, I just stared at her. I didn't have the social graces to ask how she was, her family, or any *normal* interaction. I went totally blank. She smiled with a wince, 'Oh, that's no good,' and waited for more information. But there was no thought in my brain at all, apart from '*I need to get out of here now.*'

She looked uncomfortably at her watch and said 'Okay, well I'd better go, kids are waiting for me. Take care, I'll see you soon.'

Sitting down in the safety of my car, I started to sob. My body broke apart. My good feeling about the new glasses crumbled, along with my rehab work and generally feeling better. My everything broke apart. *I was a brain cabbage, and I couldn't cope back in the real world.* I couldn't even talk to people like a normal human.

As I drove home, the road view became misty as the new glasses fogged up till I could hardly see. I wanted to die. The person who I was had gone. I'd been trying so hard to get better . . . and I wasn't! I fantasized about a passing truck taking me out of my misery.

Arriving home, I literally fell out of the driver's door. My husband ran to pick me up as my body convulsed with tears. His strong arms wrapped around me, 'Babes! Babes! What happened? What happened?' I closed my puffy eyes in pain. 'I just can't do it anymore. It's all broken.'

He led me upstairs to bed and shut the curtains (which would be his signature move for the duration of my brain injury). 'Have a sleep and you'll feel better soon; I'll keep the kids out.'

My pillow was wet by the time I drifted into slumber. *How could everyone keep loving me when I was this damaged and horrible?*

The supermarket and shopping

With a head injury, your sensitivity to noise and light is heightened. The people, the colour, the lights, the noise, are all a massive overload for a scribbled brain. If you can't get someone to do the shopping for you, then here are some suggestions:

- Use an online shopping platform
- Do only a small list so your time in the environment is limited
- Wear a cap, clear silicone ear buds, sunglasses (or tinted glasses)

- Use Google review function that shows the quietest times to shop

REINING IN CONTROL

I knew at a deep level that I was currently so different from who I was. The ability to make small talk had been deleted, and I felt safe only with my immediate circle. As friends came out to visit over the next two weeks, I found my brain scrambling for the nearest fire exit. Yet underneath it all (focussing on my why), I was determined to not be a victim. I'd had enough months of rubbing the strings on the mini violin.

Determined to beat the brain injury, I designated myself back onto school pickup and fired all my help. I took back the cleaning, the cooking, the children. I felt convinced that if I did *more*, I would get *stronger*.

I was assessed by a neuropsychiatrist, who noted my *boom/bust mentality*. I guess I was in the boom phase, because the moment I started to feel like a victim I started to get angry and do more. The neuropsychiatrist predicted I would be healed by December 2020 (five months away), but I thought *I'll show him*, and dug my heels into the ground for faster success.

I raced around the house cleaning, exercised more, did more with the kids and did more rehab. The therapists would show up and I would exclaim how good I was feeling. But behind the scenes, my mental health was on a militant slide to turmoil.

My husband became the piñata. The more I did, the more I would call him lazy; the more I yelled at him, the less he wanted to be home, so the less he was home, and the more I would moan to my friend who was living with us, or my parents who visited weekly.

I was booming and mentally busting. I was becoming toxic and my relationship with my friend who was still living with us became an opportunity to deepen the rift in my marriage. Everything seemed to be my husband's fault: *the reason for my life being torn apart; why I had lost my job; why I couldn't manage my life.* Not Covid-19 destroying our tourism business, nor the fact that a major head knock had turned my brain sideways, nor anything else. Just the husband's fault.

He wasn't the only wounded soldier in my path – I was even getting angry at my friend who was staying. Her music was too loud, I couldn't listen to her day without getting frustrated. My parents would get their heads bitten off when they commented 'You look tired.'

I was out for blood, and whoever stepped into my path was down for a massacre. I don't need you; you haven't helped me at all (what a joke). I'm going to DO IT ALL MYSELF. Boom! The pot was on the boil.

🧠 *Boom to bust in mental health*

The highs and lows of mental health are deeply connected to our basic health. When we feel good, we do more. When we feel low, we do less. It is natural to want to expand during times of success. Yet with a brain injury we are working with faulty electrical parts, and the boom phase can deplete us very quickly, leading to a bust.

On the good days, there may be a tendency to not do the rehab exercises, avoid rests, skip meals, and do a lot more than you normally would. What I experienced was that after a boom day, I would be stuck back in bed for two days in pain. Or the mental health symptoms of anxiety, anger and depression would quickly implode.

Planning and pacing, even on the good days, is best practice for rehabilitating fully. On the good days ensure you eat well, exercise and rest. These become non negotiables even as your brain heals. The rest periods will decrease, yet adding in quiet moments of meditation will be a lifetime panacea for the brain.

🧠 *Watch out for 'piñata' syndrome*

During your recovery it is easy to blame those around you for not 'understanding' the journey. The truth of the matter is that nobody knows how it feels to live through your experience unless they have been there themselves. Yet it is also not their fault. Blaming others will only create anger or hurt, which is damaging to your brain. Negative thoughts and speech will only drive people away from you.

A gift which may help is to consciously notice what the people in your life are doing for you. Take note of who is trying to help you and say thank you more. Gratitude is a superpower for mental health.

Your brain is like a GPS system

Have you ever wanted something, and suddenly you notice it everywhere? This is because of the reticular activating system (RAS) in your brain, which helps filter out irrelevant or unimportant stimuli and directs your focus toward things that matter. It's what allows you to concentrate on a specific task or conversation while tuning out background noise.

Just like a camera, what you focus on imprints a pattern in your brain. This can be thoughts, words, emotions or events. It is important for you to be aware of this. If you constantly look for the negative, your brain will look for more evidence. If you repeat a negative thought about yourself or someone else, you will manifest behaviour that validates your beliefs, and this has been scientifically proven with brain scans.

Dr Amen has shown the power of both gratitude and negative thought through SPECT (Single Photon Emission Tomograph) scans. Gratitude radiates beauty into the brain, while negative thoughts cause a lack of blood flow.

When you are going through your brain injury, the power of your thoughts and words should not be underrated. Your language towards yourself, the outside world and those you care for need to be cleaned up. This ties back into what you are inputting into your brain computer in the forms of television, social media and the conversations you have with others.

A useful tool is to put your thoughts and speech through three filters:

- Is this true?
- Is this useful?
- Is this kind?

When you start appreciating the small things in yourself and others, your brain will respond positively. A major win for mental health.

BOOM AND BUST

On the 25th of August 2020 I sent a letter to my rehab team. After nearly three months of therapy, I felt things weren't much better. Even though I was at the time comparing it to 'who I was before the accident'.

'Hi ladies, I'm sending this through as I couldn't articulate it beforehand. On waking, I have pressure at the base of my skull, sensitivity to noise (kids, TV, cutlery, the radio), and light is a total issue (even indoor lights need to be off). By 1.00pm I'm fatigued, and pressure is increasing at the base of the neck. By 3.00pm, there's tension type pressure on the temples and back of the neck. In the evening, pressure ache at the top of the neck and side temples (like there's too much blood) and heat. Eyes are tired. Light, noise and other mammals make it worse.

When driving I need to concentrate intensely, and I work a left turn route, so I don't have to cross intersections. I've discussed this with the husband tonight, as I really feel that the constant talking and listening (from people being here) and managing the kids is part of the fatigue/symptoms. The last three weeks have been all about the kids. Driving again, kids' sports, managing the household. I haven't had time for me. I think if I can learn to schedule more of the brain break alone time and quietness, it will help.

My goals are to feel like I can function normally again in society – to be around other people with noise and light not being a major issue; to get well and strong so I can give back and help others who are going through a health journey.

Concussion specialists talk a lot about 'triggers'. You rate the intensity of your symptoms from 0-10 (10 being the worst) and start to look at patterns of behaviour or symptoms that indicate the concussion flow-on is getting worse. The dirty socks on the floor at the beginning of the day aren't an issue, but by 6.00pm you are ready to murder the culprit. In the morning the fridge humming is just a background noise, but at some point it becomes a full-on concert of destruction, and you are ready to unleash Armageddon on whatever crosses your path.

The triggers – the patterns – the symptoms, that only you and those closest to you see. *And you need to slow down to see them.* If you're going fast, you don't see them, and then you crash. Boom . . . bust . . . it was coming.

I was starting to isolate everyone, and I felt as though it was working. When I started feeling frustrated and angry, it propelled me to work harder. I felt more empowered if I could say 'Screw you. I can do this on my own.'

Diary entry: *Saw the psychologist today and feel empty. I don't want to talk. I want peace, silence, and noiseless bliss.*

I felt as if it was everyone else's fault, and I was the only one who could fix it. I was listening to my meditation, exercising daily, eating right and I had whiteboard routines and lists for miles. I had this, one hundred per cent. I had taken my power back – or so I thought.

But when the anger stopped and the momentum slowed down, I lost my marbles, again at my husband. It was on a Saturday afternoon and my friend was out of the house. The kids were upstairs watching a movie and my husband could see I was frustrated, so much more than frustrated, in fact about to go psychopath at a million miles an hour. I was burnt out from the militant focus, and I was seeing mess everywhere, mess I had no control over.

I started to throw things around the room – clothes, cutlery, papers on the bench – whipping up a storm within the home.

'Calm down Katie,' as he tried to hold me still to stop me from trashing the place. I flailed wildly, ripping his arms off me and screamed 'Screw your calm down! I've had enough!'

I was tired of feeling like a broken toy in the cupboard; tired of seeing my children look at me with scared eyes; tired of my mother avoiding me (she had stopped coming over); and my mother-in-law avoiding me (she had stopped coming too); and my father telling me he didn't know 'what he would get' when he turned up at the house. I was tired of the pain in my skull, tired of rehab that felt worthless, and tired of recounting to my husband all the reasons I was tired. I was tired of my friend living with us and the conversations about me just needing to 'leave your husband and everything will be better'.

I was tired of creating balloons in my head and having them pop.

I was tired of having to stop the soothers that I enjoyed: the whiskey, the coffee, the tobacco, the chocolate. It felt like things would never be better again. I was done trying.

I screamed, as my husband looked at me like a wild animal in a zoo. I ripped my new glasses off my face and broke them into two pieces, throwing them onto the floor in a rage. Then I started to punch myself in the head screaming 'AAAAAAAAAH', over and over again and totally out of control.

Suddenly I bolted out of the back door, running first in one direction, then in another, like a wounded beast that had ravaged a village and was escaping the gunshots. Ending up hiding down in our gully by a tree stump, I felt invisible. Heavily panting, I could hardly suck air into my lungs. No one could see me from the house as the damp earth sunk into my trousers. I cowered, sobbing, unable to stop the streams of tears cascading down my hot cheeks.

I hit my head with my fists time and time again while tearing at my hair in the hope I could lift my skull off and find peace. 'Enough, enough, enough,' I whispered. 'God, please, please help me. Please help me God. Take me – take me now, I can't do this anymore. I've had enough.'

Above on the hillside I could hear my children calling for me and my husband yelling, but I remained silently hidden while rocking gently back and forth with my eyes shut. Rain clouds passed over and droplets merged with my tears as birds started flying back to their nests. I continued rocking in the dirt.

Eventually all the voices faded as the rain grew heavier and my breathing slowed. I had come back into my body and could see again. I picked at the bark on the ground, watching ants tirelessly trek homeward before dark. The sky above cracked and hollered, and I wished it would swallow me whole, evaporate me into nothing, to be free from this brain cage.

Closing my eyes, I took a breath, knowing what I had to do. Walking back inside our home to hold my husband and children for what I knew would be the last time. I'd made my *final* decision. I apologised for my tantrum and told them how sorry I was and how much I loved them.

🧠 *Rage attacks*

This may not be relevant for everyone, but anger can be a major part of concussion. The key is understanding that these mental health attacks are a result of brain dysfunction. You may be tired, you may have done too much that day, you may not have eaten properly. Your basic needs for brain health are not being met. I liken it to a power board. When we connect too many plugs into the board, the circuits can overload and explode. For the people around you, these moments are extremely hard not to take personally. When we rage at our loved ones, it is damaging to our relationships. The key is to have a health and safety plan in place for the household. This may include:

- An agreement *before the rage attacks happen* on what actions will be taken. Will you go to the cupboard alone with your noise-cancelling headphones, and do deep breathing while listening to quiet music? Will you go for some exercise? Could you have a warm shower? Put the plan in place and practise when you are feeling well.
- Understanding that you are hurting, yet you don't want to hurt them too. All the brain needs is rest.
- Communicating before you hit boiling point that you are feeling 'triggered'. This is where the traffic light system (in triggers) may help. As soon as you get to 'orange', or

your closest friends see you moving into 'orange', there needs to be a brain bath. Catch the ambulance before you are at the bottom of the cliff.

- If you are a parent, plan what the children will do if this happens. Let them know that the 'tantrum' is not about them and it is your brain having an electrical short circuit.

- Plan ahead for everyone in the household so everyone can take a safe space if this occurs.

Chapter 10

Spirituality – held by something higher

'The word is very near to you, in your mouth, and in your heart, that you may do it. See, I have set before you this day, life and good, death and evil, blessings and cursings. Choose life.' Deuteronomy 30:14,15,19

Earlier in the month I'd read a book about a secret lake that is important to the local Indigenous people for healing. Every year there is a pilgrimage to cleanse the body of negativity. I had made the final decision to go to this lake and wash off a necklace I had planned to leave for my three-year-old daughter, so that she had something beautiful to remember me by. I did not plan to return.

The day after my psychotic episode, the family left for school and work. I packed the truck with all my medication (a large satchel of antidepressants, pain killers, ADHD and migraine pills). In the back was a sleeping bag, goodbye letters to my husband and children, a few warm clothes, a bottle of whiskey to wash down the poison and a pouch of cigarettes. I sat on the couch with my coffee, completely numb.

I texted my parents and told them how much I loved them and my husband to say sorry for all I had put him through. I texted my few remaining friends to thank them for the support they had given me. Then I turned my phone off.

My loving husband had fixed my glasses that I had smashed the evening before, so for the first time in six months I drove my car out of town in complete silence.

For two hours to the destination, I was in a cocoon of nothing. No thoughts, just the soothing melodic waves of white lines. I had decided this was the end, and nothing around me, nor before me, nor behind me could get me to change that. I was completely still inside myself.

When I arrived at the deserted carpark, I turned on my phone, but there wasn't any cellphone reception. I was alone. I was numb.

All I wanted was to clean the necklace so that I could leave it for my daughter as a gift to remember her mother, then return to the vehicle to end everything.

As I approached the track, there was a fork in the path. To the left a smooth dirt track, or the one towards the right which was overgrown. I decided to take the right path as I didn't want to stumble on any stray humans who may disturb my peace.

Scrambling through brambles, with eyes firmly down on the track, I wrestled over plants, my shoes crunching in the bracken. A little black bird started to follow, flitting from tree to tree. The body was moving but my spirit felt as if it was tethered above me by a balloon string. Floating off into the eternal silence that was eminent.

I couldn't see the water because of the dense bush, and as tears rolled down my face I became anxious I would never find access to clean the necklace. After 15 minutes of walking, I found a small wooden bridge, where I lay down to stare up at the blue sky. Birds were singing, the wind softly rustling in the trees, and the smell of a crisp spring morning was filling my senses. Yet I was so tired of fighting everything, fighting the demons inside my brain since the concussion.

It seems easier to go. I'm not getting better and I'm hurting everyone. My brain is broken, and no matter what I do, I destroy everyone around me. Everyone would be better off without me.

I rolled onto my stomach, to stare at the water below the bridge. Tears flowed down my face staining the old wood as the sun danced in the water underneath me. *Enough is enough.* I tried to dangle the necklace into the water below, but the cord was four inches shy of touching, so I picked myself up to find the water and knew that it was time.

As I walked further down the path, suddenly I came across three rocks leading down to the lake's edge. *Three rocks, just like the original injury: one to trip on, one to bash my knee on, and one to smash my temple. Three rocks.*

I stepped down onto the third rock and squatted on a cold stone with my head low. As in an old movie, I started to play back scenes in my head, contemplating my life. Family, friends, the memories, and what a putrid mess things were in. One by one, I said my goodbyes to each of my beloveds, as if casting flowers onto my impending grave. Then I reached into the cold crisp lake and lovingly caressed it over my necklace. Cleansing the past so my daughter could wear it without pain.

But then, as the water touched the necklace, suddenly I heard a loud voice as clear as day.

'**LOOK UP!**'

I quickly looked around as though someone had caught me in the middle of the plan. There was no one there.

The voice came again. '**LOOK UP!**' Yelling inside my head.

As I looked up, my breath was taken away.

Framed in my view was a glorious mountain. I hadn't noticed it before. In all her glory, covered with snow, she was framed by a bluebird sky. Then as if nature was creating a majestic display, I saw birds dancing in and out of the water, and dappled light sparkling across the lake like a thousand fireworks. As I held the necklace in the water, light seemed to trace towards me and fill the inside of my body.

The voice came again, loud and clear.

'You are at the bottom; the only way is up. Keep looking up.'

My head had been so low that I hadn't realised how close the mountain was in all its magnificence, as though I could reach out and touch it. I felt a warmth glide through my body like melted honey on hot toast, along with something inside of me that I hadn't felt in a long time – love.

A fog lifted in my mind, and I had an amazing realisation: *things could not get any worse than they were right now.* I was at the complete bottom of my soul. Despite all this 'help' I was still wanting to check out of the hotel and plummet into darkness.

All the medication and rehab, *and I still wanted to end my life.* All of this 'support' and I still didn't want to be here. So, was the medication working? Was the rehab working? Or did I need *something else?*

A jolt of electricity ran through me, and I decided there and then that I had to stop everything that wasn't helping my brain. The pills, the caffeine, the alcohol, the junk food, the bad thoughts, the useless conversations, the laziness, the anger. The clarity of purpose was intense.

My ultimate fear was '*Who am I underneath all of this? Who am I underneath my "condition", my depression, my anger, my pain?'* **The me that is *now*, not the me that was**.

And I thought at that moment, sitting by the lake in view of the snow-coloured mountain: the person I am now can't be any worse than wanting to kill myself. I sat and began to pray.

I prayed for guidance. I had never been religious before (I believed in energy), but the voice was so strong in my head that it felt as if someone was right there on the rock, arms wrapped around me, whispering the same words. '**You are at the bottom; the only way is up. Keep looking up.'**

Miraculously, after ten minutes of intense prayer, my phone started to buzz with notifications (and I swear on my children's lives that there had been no service moments before).

Text messages from my parents, my husband and my friends. A voice message from a client who I had not spoken with in years needing my help. I started to cry again. A blanket of grace wrapped around me. I was loved. I was needed. I only had one direction to go. I was at the bottom of my soul, and the only way was up. ***Keep looking up***.

As I floated back to the truck, I saw a rubbish bin near where I was parked. I got all the medication and my goodbye letters and threw them away.

As I drove home, an intense peace filled my body. *Keep looking up*. ***Keep looking up***.

When I walked through the door, I ran to the couch and held my family close. My husband, my three-year-old daughter and my seven-year-old son intertwined like vines of love. Tears crept solidly, as I felt an intense surge of gratitude for being given another chance to feel their loving arms again.

Children tucked into each side, and my husband holding my hand firmly, I realised they still loved me. I'm OK. Despite all I had put them through, they were still here. ***Keep looking up***. The only thing that was important now was my family. I had to do everything in my power to heal for *them*.

Faith

Many years ago, as a natural health therapist, I had a client who was a Christian who said to me 'Katie, who is your God? I explained it was an 'energy', as I had treated religion like a buffet – take a bit of this and that from every religion and then settle on nothing. Then he said, 'How is this energy for you?'

After he left, it rattled me. Rattling my bones for years, as although I felt I could give energy to others through healing, but I had never felt a connection to a source for *me*. I would 'pray' or try 'manifestation', yet daily I felt disconnected from any sort of higher power for myself.

Like a mobile phone without a plug to charge, my energy would run out, and I would need to rest in my healing work. Yet when this voice emerged, my life changed. I tangibly felt held. I knew then that there is something greater than ourselves. Just like electricity, the unseen power that moves our spirit is here, even if we can't see it.

I have heard this voice since that day. It is a daily comfort. I talk, pray and give thanks for the small things in life. It was the final piece of the puzzle, as I had been working on the physical and mental through the rehabilitation yet had had no spiritual connection.

Having faith when life is at rock bottom is an incredible tool. The feeling of being held by something higher. Held by the energy that is in every living thing. When there is only yourself, and life is bad, there can be little hope. With faith, there is a sense of being held as you heal . . . there is hope beyond your human hands.

Also, you have a 24/7 counselling service to God (whatever your version is), where you can talk about your thoughts.

Connecting with a spiritual practice (like meditation and prayer) can bring you a sense of community and peace. Always remember we are an energetic body in a physical one, connecting to a higher 'power' can be a life saver for your mental health.

Remember how far you've come

Knowing your darkest hour is a superpower. My lowest point was driving to the lake about to take my life. When we have a frame of our rock-bottom moment, we can use this as leverage to see the truth in our progress. You may not feel as if you are healing, yet using the 'darkest hour' as a tool, you will see that you are getting better. It may be slow growth in the dirt, yet all seeds take time to root and shoot.

How you can create a spiritual practice
An easy way to start is to set your alarm 15 minutes before you would normally wake up. When lying in bed go through the following practice in your mind:

1. Give thanks for your health and your family, and add in small things you are grateful for right now. Gratitude is the foundation of prayer.
2. Apologise for any errors you feel you have made.
3. Ask for guidance and support for the day ahead.
4. If you have a spiritual text, you may set aside time reading.

Another practice I implement daily (at the end of the day) is the ancient Hawaiian healing method of Ho'opono'ono. This helps me to clear out any negative feelings I have accumulated so that I sleep better.

My version is a little different from the original, but it works:

1. Imagine the person who may be triggering negative emotions in you as though they are standing before you in your mind.
2. In your mind silently say what you need to say to let go.
3. Imagine a cord of connection between you and that person and start to flood the cord with light.

4. Repeat the Ho'opono'ono prayer (speaking on behalf of the creator – not yourself. Repeat: 'I'm sorry, please forgive me, I love you, thank you', whilst flooding the light towards them.
5. When you feel the process is complete, cut the cord and imagine the person being carried away in a ball of light.
6. Flood the area the cord was connected into your body with light.
7. Repeat 'I am healing, I am at peace.'

The 'please forgive me' be a sticking point for some people as they feel they have nothing to 'say sorry for', and this may be true, the other person may have hurt you a lot.

The premise is that 'hurt people hurt people' and the prayer is almost saying "I'm sorry you were hurt too". But if it feels unnatural to say the Ho'opono'ono prayer, just repeat "I release you" then when you are ready cut the cord.

Chapter 11

Relationships (healing rifts)

'Adapt yourself to the life you have been given, and truly love the people with whom destiny has surrounded you.' Marcus Aurelius

I came out of the planned suicide attempt with a new perspective and a few crutches that I had been abstaining from previously. I started smoking again (briefly) and enjoyed it, and managed only three weeks off my ADHD medication before I felt as if things were wobbling and I couldn't focus. But the antidepressants and the pain medication remained out of the house.

My new perspective had enlightened me that I didn't need to be perfect, and I never was. It was time to work on healing the broken parts of my life – not just my brain.

My husband and I listened to a marriage podcast together to see if we could find our way back from the violent fighting, the risk of divorce and the wedge that the injury had driven between us.

The most memorable story talked about was the 'fox' and the 'hedgehog'.

The wily fox performs all sorts of tricks to get to the hedgehog, yet the hedgehog just does one thing – it tucks up into a ball. In a relationship, we may try many different approaches to heal the rift: date nights, counselling, books, endless conversations on the couch. Just like the fox, we try lots of tricks to heal, yet the point of the story was that in a marriage, be the hedgehog. The one thing that will save the relationship is love. Love on both sides. If you love someone – just do that.

I asked my husband after we listened to the show, 'Do you love me?' He nodded, taking my hand and saying, 'Do you love me?' My eyes exploded with tears. 'Yes, yes I do love you.' He smiled, "Then let's start again.'

The walls of my heart came down, not only because I knew that he loved me, but after everything he was still willing to start again. The power of love.

With this new 'love' perspective, I started to realign my daily goals. Instead of having a to-do list, I would choose three things that were important to me for the next day and just do that. I started using the hedgehog mentality with my kids, and communicating when I needed a brain break. When I was grumpy, I would very quickly tell my family 'It's not you, I just need a rest.' This open communication without the emotion enabled me to get the space I needed without creating a storm in the teacup.

Relationships with others

This journey is not just yours. If you have family or friends, this journey is for all of you. The truth of a brain injury is that you will change. You may not be the person you were, but you can be different yet better. It is vital that they know where you are along each step of the way.

If you have children

Your advocate or specialist *must* explain to the children what is happening with your brain. They need to understand that the mood swings are *not about them*; to understand that Mum/Dad are going to take a 'brain break' and what that means and why. You may say 'I need a brain break because my brain is sore.' This will avoid them feeling as though it is their fault that you are emotionally out of control. Small people feel as though every mood you have is something that they have done, so it is critically important to communicate how you are feeling and why. They don't become your counsellor; you may like to use the formula of:

1. I'm feeling _____. You haven't done anything wrong.
2. I need a brain break and then I will feel better.

Another way to include them is in the rehabilitation process. Ideas for this are:

1. Throw a tennis ball back and forth to them (this helps your eye function).
2. Play a balance game, see who can balance the longest on one leg then switch.
3. Give them a pair of headphones and get them to sit in the cupboard with you and listen to relaxing music.
4. Do cross crawls standing up, seated or bear crawls on the floor. This helps to activate your brain.
5. If you are physically able to, play with them. Go for a walk, play tag, anything that will get your heart rate elevated, but include them in the journey.

Your language about the injury is very important. Tell them that every day your brain is getting better. Let your children know there is light at the end of the tunnel.

If you are unable to drive or participate in normal activities, explain to them why. Even the youngest child will react better with an explanation, and the knowledge that your inability to show up is not about them, it is because of your brain.

For your partner and family members

To create certainty in your relationships, those around you must be involved in the journey with you. It is crucial that they understand the symptoms of a brain injury and know your triggers (see resource section). It's important that whoever you live with knows the mood swings are not about them.

It may be beneficial to create a list of your triggers and symptoms (so your partner knows what to look for) and what needs to happen when you start to become symptomatic. Having a game plan will help you long-term. A useful technique that doesn't spur emotion is to get your partner to ask you how you are out of 10. How tired are you out of 10? How much does your head hurt out of 10? If it gets to 6/10 your partner knows that it is time for a brain bath. If you know triggers then you can plan. For example:

1. Talking or listening for more than 10 minutes makes me tired, therefore I will communicate this and go for a brain break
2. Driving makes me feel sick. Can you drive for now?
3. Socialising is too much; can you go on your own this time?

Communication on all levels is so vital, but the best thing your family can do is be a *physical* teddy bear. Even though your rational brain may want to 'talk' about how you are feeling, encourage family members to just sit quietly and give you a cuddle.

Remember that whoever you love did not cause this. Be the hedgehog, just love. Following the one thought that 'I love this person' will help you to use your brain bathing techniques when you are starting to get angry, rather than them being a punching bag.

A useful technique that doesn't spur emotion is to get your partner to ask you how you are out of 10. How tired are you out of 10? How much does your head hurt out of 10? If it gets to 6/10 your partner knows that it is time for a brain bath.

🧠 *Know your love language*

Knowing your love language (created by Gary Chapman) can help you with your recovery process. This can also help with creating your 'safety net' in all social interactions and relationships. The five types are:

1. Compliments – you enjoy people telling you how much you are loved or what a good job you are doing
2. Acts of service – you enjoy people doing things for you
3. Quality time – you enjoy spending time with those you love
4. Physical touch – you enjoy being hugged or massaged
5. Receiving gifts – you enjoy getting presents

It is worth understanding during your concussion journey how you feel love, so that you can communicate this to your family.

🧠 *Being quiet and being OK*

If you were a person who used to 'fill the space' with conversation, going through concussion can be a trying time. Now you may feel uncomfortable in social situations for two reasons:

1. You find it hard to think of what to talk about
2. You may be worried about saying the wrong thing

Know that there are people in the world who are quiet, and this is okay. We do not have to fill the gaps. Just like animals, we can be at peace with others without having to talk all the time. What people sense is your inner emotion versus the words. So being calm internally, knowing that you are allowed to be quiet, is a gift.

Chapter 12

Rebuilding a new future

'At the end of life, what really matters is not what we bought, but what we built; not what we got, but what we shared; not our competence, but our character; and not our success, but our significance. Live a life that matters. Live a life of love.'
Unknown

We decided to take a family holiday away from having rehab appointments without anyone else. My husband and the children needed to connect again and experience what life was like before all of this. *It was a game changer for reconnection.*

When we returned, I had firmly decided that I wanted our marriage to work. My friend had been living with us for nearly six months and she had been an incredible support during my darkest times. What I realised, though, was that as my support she was also my confidant, which incited hatred toward my husband. She would often say 'Leave him, let's move in together.' For the first part of my rehabilitation, this seemed like a valid option as I was blaming ALL my pain on my husband.

After the holiday, I was no longer willing to enter any negativity about him. I was the hedgehog. As a result, my tolerance for her being in our home waned quickly. I knew she had been incredible, yet her staying was now a roadblock to my full recovery. Our friendship went downhill. My only reasoning was that she had been the major support for me when Simon wasn't around and now that I was hedge hogging Simon, I wasn't giving our friendship the attention it once had. I just couldn't, I had only enough in my cup for my health and my family.

My friend moved out and my rehab continued to get stronger and stronger with my family day by day. I'm sure in many ways I hurt her and I'm forever grateful for her support and love, but I couldn't heal my marriage and still have the option to use the husband as a kick bag. I had to go in boots and all, or not at all. I love him and I had to get through this dark night of the soul with my marriage intact.

I stayed off the caffeine, continued the meditation, started to do more in my day and generally felt better. I was protecting my peace, and anyone who compromised it was disconnected from my life.

🧠 *Friends*

Many TBI sufferers talk about losing friends. Whether it is a filter issue or emotional regulation, the main problem is a lack of understanding about how your brain has changed. Humans are complex, but you have you noticed that a lot of interactions are negative? It may be whinging about life, commenting on the news or exchanging drama. The adult dynamic (especially the female one) is rife with connecting through negativity. It's a different story from being a child, where friendship is based on play.

To heal, it is important to have people in your circle that:

1. Understand the symptoms of a brain injury, so they know when you need to rest.
2. Understand that when you say something, or don't want to connect, it is not about them.
3. Come to the table with positivity and leave gossip at the gate.
4. Know your attention span is reduced and keep visits to a short time frame. If you can cope with only 10 minutes at this stage, they respect your brain and don't sit for hours.

5. Learn the trigger traffic light (see resource section), so they have empathy for your choices of socialisation (e.g. walk vs café).

🧠 *Create safety*

A quote that has stayed with me since my rehabilitation (then viewing my son's journey) is: *'If you want to make the world a better place, make people feel safe.'* Reflecting on how unsafe I felt during my recovery, how when I yelled at my husband, friends and my children . . . I made them feel unsafe. The guilt that followed the anger made me feel unsafe again. Would they still like me? Would they still love me? Am I worthy? This experience taught me to really try to feel safe myself and make others feel safe. We can accept someone as they are, because that negative emotion is often a sign they feel unsafe.

How can you create safety in your life? Or a better word may be 'certainty'. It is one of the major human needs. Like non-negotiables, we can start to cultivate daily habits that anchor you, and those you love, into their body to create safety. Ask yourself these questions:

1. What calms me down?
2. What makes me feel good?
3. What activities make me smile?
4. What activity feels easy and enjoyable?

Vulnerability – be cautious of who enters your circle

In the first stages of your recovery, you may be extremely vulnerable – not only emotionally but physically. It is exceptionally important to have people around you that you trust. Do not allow anyone to:

- Influence you to make life decisions
- Take up your brain space if they are negative
- Encourage them to give you money or possessions
- Control your life to their benefit

Try to keep your inner circle (including carers) to a group of people who are positive and focussed on your recovery. If you feel at any time that a person is there for their own benefit or may be trying to get you to make life-changing decisions, always get a second opinion on their behaviour.

Losing humans

The AA (Alcoholics Anonymous) maxim 'What others think of me is none of my business' is a gift for brain injury. You have changed and this may cause upset for some. Real friends will stay, fair-weather friends will go. It becomes a natural filter for those who truly care for you. Worrying about what other people think about you is indeed a complete waste of brain space. If you don't want to socialise – don't. If you don't want to engage in small talk – don't. You don't have to fill space. There are plenty of people who are comfortable being quiet, as I've said, so learn to protect your brain and set boundaries around conversation.

Those that gossip and talk negatively will drag you down. Guard your brain from those types of humans. For me, joining a church was the first step back into socialising in groups larger than two. Yet the sojourn was about parallel play versus intense interaction. Like being a child again, I started to find things I enjoyed doing, and found other humans who liked doing the same things. You may find it helpful (as you heal) that you can:

- Join a community group
- Volunteer
- Re-engage a hobby or start a new one

The natural filter

Not being able to display most of the normal social graces can be an issue with brain injuries. It is as though we cannot 'act' human any more, so often the filter may come off. We may say inappropriate things which offend, we may have little to share in filling conversations, and some days we don't want to participate at all. Know that you may be different, but you are not broken. The filter creates a net for those who love you to stay in, and like gold panning the rest of the dirt falls away. Be you and keep going.

The relationship with yourself
This journey is a heart one, not just a head one. Things that helped me:

- Cry when you need to. Crying helps to release stress from the body.
- Acknowledge that there is a natural grieving process after the brain injury. You have lost who you were. The stages of grief are denial, anger, bargaining, depression and acceptance, but not necessarily in that order, and they can repeat many times over.
- Understand you are not broken. You are different but you are not unusable. Everyone has something to offer, and you can find a new path.
- Set your boundaries firmly with other people so that when you are feeling unwell you take time out. Otherwise, you will spill emotion onto other people, it is better to be brave at the beginning.
- Celebrate the small wins.
- Do the rehab and become obsessed with helping your brain.

- Take one day at a time.
- This too shall pass – a bad day can be offset with some rest and a healthy meal.
- Create tent pegs for your day. Find three things that will anchor you (mine were exercise, meditation and nutrition).
- Don't blame others for your symptoms. If you are angry, sad, out of control or overwhelmed, take it as a sign that you need a brain break. Nobody is doing it to you, and they are on your team.

Chapter 13

Getting back into life again

'Keep going . . . you never know how strong you are until you look back at everything you've overcome. Kerry Smith

As life started to get better, I reconnected with friends I had not seen since before Covid. Because I was still getting migraines, neck and knee pain and intracranial pressure (despite six months of relentless rehabilitation), my friend suggested that I go and see a manual physiotherapist who specialised in concussion.

The concussion physiotherapist I had been seeing did little manual therapy. Seeing this new physiotherapist was an absolute game changer for recovery. Every single session I had with her would make me feel sick and I needed to go to bed, but she explained this was normal as we were stirring up the nervous system. I had acupuncture, massage and physiotherapy with someone who understood why my neck was still in so much trouble. Seeing the manual physiotherapist meant I could turn my head properly for the first time in six months, and it didn't make me want to throw up.

Manual therapy

As soon as you can, get some sort of manual therapy on your neck. 95 per cent of post-concussion symptoms involve the neck, so for healing it is crucial to address neck or spine issues. If you are seeing a neuro physiotherapist, they are primarily working with the brain, so having manual therapy as well is essential.

In the beginning, your neck may be extremely tender, so manual therapy may not be an option. Yet there are a few non-invasive strategies that can provide relief without digging into too much of the muscle pain. Some of the things that helped me during the early stages of my brain recovery (please see the resource section for more information on alternative therapies) were:

- Craniosacral therapy – a very gentle non-invasive technique to balance the nervous system
- Stretching
- Acupuncture
- Physiotherapy

As the inflammation reduced:

- Gentle massage and trigger point therapy
- Using a foam roller or tennis ball to deactivate trigger points
- A chiropractor or osteopath for deeper manipulations on the bones and muscles

HAPPINESS RETURNING

I was feeling as if things were on the up: I was planning and pacing, caffeine free, back to eating low carb, exercising every morning, and following the rules. My relationships were better, I had a relationship with God, and for the first time in months a sense of happiness was returning. So my occupational therapist suggested it was time to go back to work, 'Let's get you back into life again.'

I hadn't worked for six months, with no screen time, nor any sense of routine apart from the one I implemented. Re-entering the real world again was a daunting idea. I had lost my 'role' in our family business during Covid-19. My role had been absorbed into three other people, so I had no 'job' to return to. The return-to-work plan (which is the normal rehabilitation process here in New Zealand) was slightly skewed, as I had no work to return to. The plan was to find what the 'new' Katie could do.

I still wasn't back to three speeds of fast Katie. My memory was very bad, I was still getting headaches and fatigue, but I was a *new version of myself* – which I had accepted. The old Katie was gone, and I had to start where I was.

The rehabilitation programme organised an occupational assessment to see what I could do whilst still dealing with a recovering brain.

I was feeling perky and optimistic about this new adventure when the middle-aged gentleman arrived at home to interview me on what I felt I could do. *I requested something without too many humans, lights or noise.* The list consisted of farm assistant, shelf stacker, forestry worker, naturopath (my old job), massage therapist (old job).

I told him 'I don't think I can handle too much stress. What about those lollipop people that hold the signs on the road?' The career advisor smiled and said, 'I'll put it down and we can see what we can do.'

Then we worked on my resume. There were massive holes in my memory – I couldn't remember where I was employed and what year. He said, 'That's okay, we will work with what we have. I'll email through your resume and let's get you back to work!'

After he left I went to bed at 11.00am, exhausted with a headache, sleeping the rest of the day until the children arrived home.

The next day, inspired by the idea of getting a job, I decided to create my own resume. I was ready to get back into the world, and lo and behold in the newspaper was a PERFECT job for me: 20 hours a week and I knew the boss from when I was working in our tourism business! I felt divinely led to apply despite my ongoing symptoms.

After I prepared my presentation, I emailed the boss personally to let her know my application was on its way to her inbox. Within minutes I received an email back to ask if I was available for a phone call that day during her lunch break. *Of course, I would love to chat, I'm not busy at all.*

I sat on the armchair in my lounge for at least an hour waiting for the phone to ring. I pounced on the call excitedly at 1.00pm and the first thing I said (even before saying *'Hello, Katie here'*) was 'Have you eaten your lunch?'

After a dramatic pause on the other end of the phone, she coughed politely. 'I'm sorry?' *Obviously, she didn't hear me the first time.* 'Have you had your lunch?'

A clearing of the throat on the other end of the phone, the manager sounded confused. 'I'm sorry, I don't understand.'

Enthusiastically I launched in. 'Well, you said earlier today that you'd call in your lunch break, and I'm just making sure you've had your lunch.'

Another pregnant pause and a slight giggle. 'Yes . . . I've had my lunch, thank you.'

At this point, I sensed I wasn't sounding normal. My conversation was stilted and the brain clunking. I began overcompensating by trying too hard to appear normal. I asked questions about the role, what her vision was, what the plan was. I seemed to have turned the mood around when suddenly she had 'another meeting to get to' and the phone call was cut short.

But I was still hopeful, telling *everyone* I was going to get the job. I knew the people, had lots of connections, it would work with the kids, and I could do it standing on my head. Everyone was happy for me, because '*You know you really deserve something good to happen*'. Yes, I do deserve that, don't I, God? Don't I deserve a win after this hellish ride?

That evening, despite the roaring headache that ensued from being on the computer, I went to bed like a child before Christmas. I started planning my new life when my imaginary job offer came through. When I saw the concussion team, I told them all how I was going well and that I would be back to work very soon. I had full faith that this was my path.

To increase my stamina, each day I would do a little bit more work on the computer. Pain increased and then I developed increased peripheral neuropathy (tingling and numbness) in my right hand, so I started back on a prescription of nerve inhibitors. I couldn't risk not being able to work.

Often life doesn't work out how we think it is going to.

On the day when the 'call backs' for interviews were happening, I randomly saw an old friend at the local swimming pool that I hadn't seen since before my head knock. My children ran to play as we talked, and she dropped into the conversation that she had just got a call back for the same role I had applied for. As I listened to her talking about her 'potential new job', my heart sank. I smiled with fake enthusiasm for her, yet all the while thinking 'I didn't get a call back. They don't want me . . . because my brain is broken'.

It felt as if the ground was crashing down from underneath me. The old story resurfaced: I'm doing all this work to heal my *brain and it still isn't good enough.* Back in the carpark, the noise of my children in the back seat blurred to a dull murmur. I was in the numb place where nobody could touch me – unable to feel or hear anything.

My children asked a question which I glibly replied to, 'Okay, yep whatever.' The kids screamed Yaaay!' I hadn't heard a word they'd said, but apparently I had just committed to takeaways and a movie night. I continued to sit in the car with the kids excitedly buzzing in the back, and then and there decided to email the boss I had spoken to.

Here's the email:

'Thanks so much for considering me for the role. Just wondering if the position has already been filled as I've just seen my friend who has had a call back, and I didn't get one. I've got a few projects on the boil, so would really appreciate knowing if I haven't made the cut.'

I lied. I had no projects on the boil and was still under the rehab programme for my head injury, and I was desperate for some kind of self-esteem boost... anything to validate me. Almost immediately I received an email saying, *'Due to a high number of applicants, you are unsuccessful at this time.'* I felt numb.

The next day after my rejection, I applied for another part-time role. Twelve hours a week (perfect) teaching aqua dance to seniors. I'd worked as a personal trainer for a good chunk of my early days – easy. Again, I told everyone 'This is it! I can do this.' Got an interview, did the interview, didn't get the job.

Diary entry: *The feeling like I'm not good enough sits inside me like a cavernous wave. I'm so scared about work and what that looks like. Will anyone want me? Am I any good anymore?*

I was feeling vulnerable and small; each time I had to put myself out into society it seemed to reinforce that I had changed, and I couldn't cope with day-to-day life.

When I picked the kids up from day care and school, I would feel awkward around the other parents. When I saw my in-laws, or spoke to friends, I felt uncomfortable and self-conscious. The only people I felt entirely safe with were my children, my parents and my husband. A foreboding sensation enveloped me that the rest of the world was out to get me. And if not now, then when?

The psychologist told me this was irrational, that I should look for the positives. But the more I stepped out of my comfort zone, the more it burnt like an open wound. I felt as though the whole world could see I had changed.

With this new pressure of having to find a job, I found even the slightest change too much. If my husband's work hours changed, I got upset. If the day didn't go as planned, I'd get angry. If the kids wouldn't do as I asked, I would cry.

The problem with identifying with one part of yourself is that you risk damaging all other parts for the sake of perfection. If I didn't get the jobs I applied for, immediately I felt unwanted, like a failure. My anxiety around fitting back into the world again after the head injury hinged on this one thing – *this being wanted by someone, someone to employ me, to show me I was enough.*

The thoughts were starting to spiral me down towards the hole again. But the voice returned to my head.

'You are at the bottom; the only way is up. Keep looking up.'

Before the tears hit, I looked at my kids and thought about how far I had come. I loved them so much, and my husband. How happy my kids were, I'm a good mum. I thought of my husband and how our relationship has grown so much deeper since the head injury. The thought struck me *'I am more than my resume'.*

I knew I had put all my emotional eggs in one basket, yet a strong resolve came from it – that I was determined to never let anyone feel as low as I did again.

Suddenly with this new vulnerability I felt a revelation about how the elderly feel, how disabled people feel, how the kids felt in the classes that I never struggled in. I understood the impact of not being good enough. Being in that subset of society that didn't make straight A's, or have the perfect hair (or brain), and it made me stronger. *I didn't have to be perfect*, and I never would be again. The superwoman ideal that I was struggling for before the head knock would never be my reality again. I couldn't even cope with the supermarket.

But for the first time ever I learnt the importance of one foot in front of the other. Screw the five-year plan, screw the affirmation bull crap. My goal is to get through today with minimum impact on the people I love, and maximum impact on being a kind human.

The stages of grief

The pattern of illness is that we can constantly look back to the past and grieve over who we were – the old identity, the old you, the person that seemed to have it all sewed together. The greater you were in the past, the more severe the journey of grief can be. Grief is known to occur in five stages:

1. Denial. In concussion this may be the post-concussion stage where you start to notice issues and put it down to other things like stress.

2. Anger. We feel angry that this has happened to us. Many may think 'There is not a God' or 'Why is this happening to me?'

3. Bargaining. Where we start to try new strategies to deal with the concussion. This could be the rehabilitation phase. 'If I do this, I may feel better.'

4. Depression. We look back at who we were (because the road to recovery can be hard) and feel a deep sense of loss that we are now different.

5. Acceptance. The most powerful stage. For any diagnosis, when we start where we are, we can truly heal. Accepting that although our brain is different, growth can happen in the dirt. It may not be the flowers you expect, but a new life will come out of your journey.

Holding a funeral for 'who you were'

This may sound dramatic, but it is a process that I created during my rehabilitation. I held my own funeral for the person I was. The ultimate ceremony for letting go of expectations based on the past. I knew that to heal, I had to let the person I was go. Let go of the high-powered version of myself to find peace. The past is gone, and no matter how you try, the new version of yourself will not be the same person that you were. I wrote myself a letter and burnt it, along with some photographs that represented the old me, and knew that it was time to start creating a 2.0 version. It was time to plant a new 'seed' for the new life.

Don't put all your eggs in one basket

A tool that can be extremely powerful when you start to reintegrate into society is making a list of your achievements:

1. Where have you improved since your head injury?
2. What is going well in your life?
3. What have you learnt?
4. Who loves you?

People I have met who have gone through TBIs have talked about the discrimination from people who know what they have experienced. There is a fear of being judged because their brain works differently. By not putting all your eggs in one basket (knowing your strengths in all areas of your life) you can hold onto your self-esteem when you start looking for jobs again.

🧠 *Job hunting*

A helpful exercise is to write out the following:

1. What am I passionate about?
2. What sort of hours would I like to work?
3. What kind of environment do I want to work in?
4. What kind of values do I want the company to have?

Making it clear what you want can help you to navigate the job market. Remember that you are choosing them as much as they are choosing you. Despite your injuries, you are still capable of doing something (even if the role is smaller than you had before), and having purpose is a great way to build momentum.

🧠 *Volunteering*

Volunteering can be a fantastic way to start to integrate back into society again after your head trauma. There is no pressure to 'be' a certain way, and it enables you to be in social environments and contribute. Find an organisation that aligns with your values, and then ensure that your energy is maintained by working the hours that fit your schedule.

🧠 *Dealing with social situations*

Listening is an underrated skill in modern society, and it can be your superpower as you step back into society again. Learning to ask questions, versus answering them, can open doors for connection in situations where you feel uncomfortable. It may help to make a list of conversation questions, so that if you find yourself stuck you can revert to these questions as a default.

- What have you been doing recently?
- How is your family?
- How is work going for you?
- How's your week been?

People love to be heard and when we put ourselves in the role of questioner it is a two-way win in social situations. Then you don't have to have all the answers in a brain that may not be full of any.

On the flip side, if you find after your head injury you have a 'blabber mouth' (which can happen), learning to close it and listen is also a gift. Press your tongue to the roof of your mouth and learn to breathe deep into your belly to calm down the incessant thoughts. Really try to see the person across from you instead of interjecting when your brain starts to rattle off.

WAKE UP AND START AGAIN

Still unemployed, I would get up each day and start again. Take a breath and begin to assess what was working, what wasn't working and start again. Some days I would fight with the husband, lose my mouth with the kids, apologise, and start again the next day. I became very good at apologising for my behaviour and ensuring no one thought it was because of them.

The more time I spent on the computer the worse my headaches got, but I was determined to do something. I started researching the brain and looking at what made me happy and what didn't; what foods made me feel good and what didn't; which people made me happy and who didn't. It was all very black and white, but I was tired of working in the grey.

A head injury puts you in the mist and you can really get lost in yourself. I needed to build a glass bridge out of the chaos so with trust I put one foot in front of the other hoping to get to the other side.

My neck and knee still weren't right, but after eight months on the concussion programme I was signed off. Yet I still wasn't right physically, so the local doctor approved another six weeks until I could have a formal assessment with a specialist in the new year.

Over the Christmas period things went from a quiet life to full on entertainment schedule with the kids. Because they were off school, I went from having daily brain breaks to having no time at all on my own. Driving almost every day with the children I suddenly developed neural symptoms that I had not experienced before.

My hand would go numb when driving and I felt as if I had spiders crawling up the back of my skull. I didn't talk too much about it, just climbed into the painkillers again and carried on. My mood worsened due to not having brain breaks and it seemed like the few months of happiness were evaporating as quickly as water on concrete in the summer.

Still, because I knew I was not as low as I had been, there was an immense hardening in my spirit, and each day I got up and started again.

I was determined to use this harrowing time of my life to help others. There is only so much time that you can dedicate to yourself until you get bored. So over the Christmas break I began reading, devouring concussion information, looking at the parallels of what I had personally found worked and what was irrelevant. I got excited about the idea of going back to my first love of natural medicine and helping others to avoid the pitfalls that I was going through. I set a goal of being off the welfare system by February, even though no job was in sight.

Find a distraction

If you have a hobby or an interest, start to explore how you can get better at it as soon as possible. Staring at your own navel during recovery can be debilitating, especially if you don't feel you are getting better.

By distracting the brain with learning, you can start to unlock neural pathways that will help you to focus less on your pain and more on your project. Even if you can't see a pathway for this to become a job, remember the brain can only focus on one thing at a time, so by using this superpower you can distract yourself from constantly thinking about what hurts.

STILL UNEMPLOYED

February arrived, and I was still unemployed. The children went back to school, and I was left with pressure headaches, pressure in the back of the skull, numbness in my arm, a buckling knee, and thousands of dollars out of pocket for physio, osteopathy and therapists. I was frustrated, yet hopeful that the next 'specialist' I was booked into could give me answers for the ongoing physical symptoms.

I drove an hour on my own to see the doctor who was assessing me to see what jobs I could go back to, and whether I needed further treatment. My case manager had told me that the goal was to rehabilitate back to 'pre-injury' health, of working 30 hours per week.

When I arrived at the clinic a young receptionist led me through a locked door into the specialist's waiting room. After 10 minutes, a small Indian practitioner poked his head out of an office and barked, 'Who are you? Are you here to see me?' He looked furtively around to see if there were any other humans in the hallway.

'Yes, I am here to see you – I think?'

He blinked, adjusting the tiny wire glasses on his frowning face 'Who let you in?' he spat. 'Was she short, with dark hair?' I shrugged my shoulders.

The doctor sniffed. 'Okay, what's your name?" I told him and shutting the door he said, 'Okay, five minutes.'

I burst out laughing aloud and waited for the doctor to be ready for our appointment. Finally, seated in HIS small, overheated office, he asked me to recount the entire journey again. He did a few eye tests, looked at my head movement and balance, all of which took five minutes. He muttered 'Good . . . good . . . good', randomly scrawling notes in his white notebook. Abruptly he asked, 'Anything else?'

As I sat back down, I told him about my knee 'popping' and the constant feeling of it buckling, and the neuropathy, especially when driving (which I had already Googled and found a link between damage to the C5-C6 vertebrae). I explained about the consistent headaches and the symptoms that weren't going away.

He curled his lip after listening for a few minutes, and said 'Mrs Jolly, you are competent to return to work. I believe you are stressed, and you just need to start doing more yoga. I am signing you off to work for 30 hours a week, and I will send the report to your case manager.'

As I sat back in the car, my blood boiled vehemently for two reasons:

1. He hadn't taken the time to read my case notes and did not listen to my concerns.
2. My previous experience as a naturopath was outraged by his lack of empathy or investigative follow-up.

So I wrote a letter to his office and sent a copy to my case manager demanding an MRI on my neck to rule out damage to the vertebrae.

The squeaky wheel does get the oil as three weeks later when I had an MRI, they found annular tears in C5-C6 and a disc bulge in between these two discs, all of which produce cervical radiculopathy symptoms, which I had. Headaches, vision problems, and numbness in my shoulder, hands and biceps are all associated with this area.

Having a PhD in your own problem

Your body is a barometer that tells you when things are awry. If you can research your own issue, it will help you to navigate specialist appointments.

Know that when you see a specialist (or any practitioner), they are focussing on you for your time slot only. It is important to have a list of questions and concerns before you enter the room, so that you can get answers in that appointment time.

It is always beneficial to get a second opinion if you can if you feel that there is a deeper problem happening with your health. And don't take 'no' for an answer.

MORE REFERRALS

I was referred to yet another specialist, a leading brain and spine specialist in the country. But this time I was prepared, sending through an email with my questions, and I took my husband with me to the appointment. We travelled two hours to see him, and he was 10 minutes late (even though we were the first client). Once again, this doctor asked me to recount the entire year's story of the three rocks and all my symptoms.

He never even used my name. I was a number on his worksheet. I did a series of tests, then he sat me down, acknowledged I had a disc bulge, then commented it was 'nothing to worry about at all'. Then he shook my hand and tried to get me out the door as fast as he could. When I asked him about the numbness, he said, 'You need to meditate, do some yoga, and relax. It will heal in time.' We were promptly ushered out the door.

We had driven two hours to see this man, after a year of hell recovering from the brain injury. I did a four hour round trip to hear him say 'Don't worry, do yoga'.

I burst out laughing in the car. My husband was confused. 'Are you happy? Good result?' I laughed hysterically again. 'We've driven all this way for him to tell me to do more yoga – which I already do – and he didn't tell me why any of my symptoms are still there. I've got a Google PhD in the C5-C6 disc issue, I know that's why I'm getting the symptoms, and he's dismissed me like I'm a teenager with a zit on a date.'

'What would you have liked to have happened?' my husband asked.

I fumed: 'Read the case notes, arsehole, and use my name. Explain to me what the MRI means and tell me why the symptoms are happening and what I can do to fix them. That's all!'

My husband reached for my hand, 'Well at least you don't have to have surgery.' As a Naturopath with an understanding of the health system, I decided to email my questions to the clinic. A stoic reply ensued to say that the doctor was purely employed for an accident compensation assessment (to see whether I could work again). So I wrote a letter back:

'Thank you so much for your response. I would like to give you some feedback to pass on to the doctor if you wouldn't mind. During the appointment, he had not read my case notes nor used my name. My questions were left unanswered, and I think it would be best practice for further clients if you realise that you are not living the lives of the 'numbers' on your worksheets. We are not numbers – we are people, with families and feelings, who want to get better. We are not a list of "symptoms" that you tick in boxes. In the future, I hope you treat people with the dignity they deserve when they are navigating their health problems.'

That week I complained to my physio about the specialist and the fact that a year later my neck and knee still weren't right. She blinked. 'What – your knee still isn't right? We've been working so much on your neck and back that I totally forgot about your knee. What's wrong with it again?'

To be totally fair, I had only mentioned it in the first session, and in the meantime we had been working on the neck issues for months.

Immediately I was referred for an MRI. They found a torn meniscus and grade 111, something else with a Baker cyst (a fluid-filled growth behind the knee) and something else that showed I shouldn't have been running during my rehabilitation at all. Months of aching legs and painkillers, and they finally found the reason. Keyhole surgery was prescribed. The last puzzle pieces were put into place.

Intuition

Nobody else is living inside your body. If you feel that something is off and the advice, medication or treatment is not working, do not be scared to push back on specialists to find answers. Most practitioners are working from a 'book' of symptoms, or experience in other people's journey. Do not forget your inner voice in this process, and always ask questions when you feel that treatment is not working for you.

Advocacy within the system

When you are dealing with the health system, most of the time you are a number. If you realise this then it is easier to navigate the journey. For all appointments:

1. Prepare questions before you attend.
2. Make a list of your current symptoms, so that you can ask questions.
3. If you can, research your symptoms so that you understand what may be causing the problem.
4. Always take an advocate with you who can be your voice if suddenly you get overwhelmed during the appointment.
5. Ask for bloodwork and further investigation to find the 'why'.
6. If your medication is not doing its job, tell your practitioner. If you suddenly develop new symptoms, or those you have do not abate with medication, tell your practitioner.

Chapter 14

Finding your place

'A house is made of bricks and beams. A home is made of hopes and dreams.' Ralph Waldo Emerson

It was March 2021, almost a year since the concussion, and I was ready to get back into society again. Regular exercise, clean eating and rehabilitation was automated, and I prayed that the perfect job would appear – and it did. I had decided to return to Natural Health, inspired by what I had learnt about the brain.

I was nervous when interviewed for a job with a non-government organisation for a health coach role. I wanted to be wanted. Divine timing intervened and finally I received a job offer. The pay was a lot less than I had been paid in years, yet being employed was a gift on so many levels.

The actual work was very easy (from years of working as a naturopath) and it gave me purpose in the morning. In the first few weeks, the stress of getting out of the door was immense, because I was so used to being able to swan through my day when the children were at school. I had to be extremely disciplined about preparing my food, organising the children, fitting in my exercise in order to make it through the day well.

But months of living like an army cadet served me well because the routine of work created another structure in our lives. I would return from work happy having helped other people, although exhausted. I was able to be my authentic self, in an industry I loved. During the first part of employment, I would go to bed extremely early, and my headaches returned.

What I learnt, however, is that every new change could potentially reignite symptoms, and it was only time that would support the brain expansion. The role was working with people who also had health issues, so it enabled me to step outside of my own story and support others. I could also use my mental health journey and the rehabilitation lessons as a pivotal tool to teach other people how to navigate through their own issues. I was able to be authentic in my interactions. People felt like they weren't alone and that 'perfect' wasn't a goal, progress was more important.

I found on days when I ate badly, my symptoms would resurface. The days when I chose not to exercise (when I was sitting down at a computer for a lot of the time) resulted in headaches. When I had to drive a 90 minute roundtrip to a neighbouring town, I would get aches in my body like the original injury. A pattern emerged of how my lifestyle impacted my health.

The symptoms resurfacing were a beautiful reminder that the rehab journey works, and it is ongoing. Looking at the 'why' and knowing the 'what' can help reinforce permanent lifestyle changes.

But as fate would have it after just eight weeks of working, my son suffered a bad concussion and was signed off school for six months.

His moods were insatiable, and we spent a lot of time together in dark cupboards. However, this time, rather than falling victim to needing everybody else to 'fix' him, I did the work alongside the specialists.

I changed his diet, did the rehab alongside him, and held him close when the brain went haywire. I witnessed again the emotional instability of the brain being injured. But because of my own journey, I was able to understand where he was, and rather than entirely relying on the specialists, I was able to support his rehabilitation journey.

Although my son was the most important thing in my life at that time, I knew for myself I needed to have some kind of work distraction, separate from the problems. I contacted the non-government organisation who had employed me as the health coach and suggested I could create a workplace health programme for the staff, using my naturopathy, nutrition and fitness skills to help the people who were helping others. I could work two days onsite and the rest of the time I would support my son. They agreed, and I was able to find a balance between my family and work, for the first time ever.

For two years I worked for the organisation, first helping those in the community, then creating a wellness programme for the staff, serving up to 14 clients in a day with diverse health issues. And the superpower of the concussion journey was that every person who walked in the door I understood, because I too had been there emotionally. The foundations of who I was 'before' the injury, had found a beautiful ikigai (a sense of purpose and reason for living).

The brain is just like a muscle

In the gym when you build a muscle encouraging it to be stronger, there will be a period of adjustment and pain. Likewise, when you start to add more things into your daily routine (like starting work again), the brain can hurt. By knowing this is normal, you can start to expand your experience of life.

The pain is not a sign to stop, it is a sign that your brain is growing again. Yet during these growth moments, it is important to hold tight to the practices, ensure you get a good sleep, eat well and exercise.

Finding your ikigai

This is an exercise that may help you navigate 'how' to get back into life again:

- Write out all your interests. What are you passionate about?
- What did you do before the injury that feels easy to you if you were to do it again?
- How can any of these skills help others?
- List jobs that align with the first three questions.

Being authentically you

Perfection is a complete myth and when we feel 'less than' we can create a barrier between ourselves and other humans by trying to be someone else. Everyone has a fear of 'not being enough'; everyone struggles with something. As my mother says, 'Everyone has a cross to bear' and knowing this can be a gift to help you to step outside your own story to connect with other people. You may not move into an industry where you are helping other people, but knowing that everyone has the same basic fear can free you from feeling 'different'.

The superpower of compassion

It may not feel like a superpower right now, but you have been given the gift of human empathy. You understand what it feels like to not 'be enough', to understand pain and the discomfort of feeling socially awkward. You understand 'fear' of not being in control and how it feels to forget things. You understand anger, depression, anxiety and the whirlwind of emotions that sit inside the brain.

This knowledge is a superpower, because everything you have been through, many other humans have a similar experience. From our journey we can start to understand all the subsets of society who often feel similar and empathise not judge.

The law of reciprocity

I stared at my navel for over a year, searching for what was wrong with me and why. Yet when I started to help others, it created a distraction from my own problems. Because the brain focuses on whatever we think, if we constantly focus on the problems, the problems are what we'll constantly see in front of us. When we give, in the form of our time or attention, we also receive. Contribution is a powerful lever to help your self-esteem.

An exercise that may help is:

Write on a piece of paper all the ways that you can give back, even if you are bedridden now or feel like you have nothing to give. Examples may be:

- I can listen to my partner talk about their day
- I could make a nice dinner for my family
- I can write a poem to give away
- I can volunteer for a local organisation
- I could go for a walk and pick up trash as I go

Returning to work

Returning to work reinforced the idea of having daily non-negotiables. We can't control the outside world, and there are going to be some days when you feel worse than others. The non-negotiables are the list of things that every day help you to feel grounded.

Imagine you are on the side of a mountain trying to pitch a tent. You must drive the tent pegs into the ground to keep the fabric in place. When the wind blows (life) we are stable. When the rain comes (emotion or symptoms reappear), we have routine and stability to hold us in place. Focusing on controlling the controllables is a great way to stop the tent flying off the mountain. I have found it powerful to choose three 'tent pegs' that I practice daily, which help with my ongoing brain health:

1. Exercise daily – to get oxygen into the brain
2. Pray/Meditate – to calm the brain down and focus
3. Eat a clean diet – to fuel the brain for optimum performance

I started working back in the health industry as a health coach and then my own son had a bad concussion a few months later, as explained earlier, so I had to leave and help with his rehabilitation for six months. But this time, rather than falling victim to needing everybody else to 'fix' him, I did the work alongside the specialists. I witnessed again the emotional instability of our brain being scrambled, yet I knew *how* to help him, because I had walked out of the dirt.

Then as he healed, I formulated a workplace health programme for the original company I had started working for, helping up to 14 clients a day. And the superpower of the concussion journey was that every person who walked in the door I understood, because I too had been there emotionally.

Every experience I have had in my lifetime seemed to converge together to focus on brain health. The years of studying, the mental health journey prior to my concussion, then moving from being injured to helping my son through a similar path.

Noticing these 'life' patterns led me further and further into studying brain health, eventually to study as a Brain Health Trainer with Dr Amen. Everything reinforced the importance of our brain. *Because when we lose something, we know its value.*

Look for the lesson

In life if we look for the lesson in all situations, we can learn and grow. Rather than feeling like a victim of our circumstances, we can look for patterns to see common themes and take the message out of the mess. Good things happen, bad things happen. Sometimes there is not a clear lesson except that it makes you stronger. Often we can't rationalise the pain, yet by looking for the gift in the grind, we build grit.
Growth happens in the dirt.

Epilogue – You are not broken

'In the infinity of life where I am, all is perfect, whole and complete. I see any resistance patterns within me only as something to release. They have no power over me. I am the power in my world. I flow with the changes taking place in my life as best I can. I approve of myself and the way I am changing. I am doing the best I can. Each day gets easier. I rejoice that I am in the rhythm and flow of my ever-changing life. Today is a wonderful day. I choose to make it so. All is well in my world.' Louise Hay

A run in the bush changed my life. All I can really remember is being airborne, my head hitting a rock and my son screaming in the distance. Somehow I got up, as we all do, and continued with my day without any memory of the experiences I had recorded on my phone.

Being diagnosed with a head injury is scary, not just for yourself but for those closest to you. There are ones who can see you are not who you once were, but there are others who will never understand why you've disappeared from social media, or have said the wrong thing, or don't even want to talk some days.

The years of growth have been exceptional: from not being able to drive for four months, write properly or even piece together a sentence some days, to today where my life is dedicated to helping others out of the mud.

Some days I slept in the cupboard and cried in the cupboard. Some days the anger overtook me, or I sat with nothing in my head at all.

I would walk into rooms not knowing why I was there or be so frustrated with the change in my brain that I wanted to rip my head off. Sometimes I would see people and not be able to make conversation, feeling naked, vulnerable, and completely inadequate in the real world.

A person with a brain injury can look completely normal. Like so many other illnesses that are on the inside, you don't receive the same empathy because it's not a visible thing. It's not a broken limb, it's a broken brain.

Years on, my injury doesn't define me anymore. It is a story to hopefully help others heal. At some point, looking around and realising that everyone has a cross to bear, has brought me to a new sense of belonging. Perfect doesn't exist – and that's okay.

The important part of growth is just getting up every day and trying again. When you are at the bottom and think you can't get any lower – trust me you can. But eventually you'll decide that it's time to swim upwards. Only you can make that choice, no one else – no pill, no therapist, no amount of money or opportunity. Only you... you are the anchor that sinks yourself, and the buoy that floats you. *Some days you just need to decide which you are going to be.*

People pay good money for manure to plant their prize roses in, and life is just like that. Out of the muck, you can grow into an awesome human being. Keep pruning the dead heads (the parts of life that don't serve you), raise your face to the sun, and take out everything that doesn't serve you to nuture the best version of the new you. **There is growth in the dirt.**

As I write this today, my marriage is thriving, and my children are happy. I no longer worry about what people think of me, and I am qualified to help people with their own brain health journey. My journey into brain health allowed me to wean off countless medications. As I focus daily on what helps the brain, and avoid what harms it, my life has become filled with deeper connections to others. I am grateful for just being alive.

What the experience taught me has marked my path for life:

1. *Love the people who support and love you for who you are, warts and all.*

2. *Life is short and if you live your life waiting to be perfect, you will miss out.*

3. *What you think about, watch and choose to associate your mind with shapes your world. Be discerning about your thoughts, words and actions and what you allow into your brain space. Focus on positivity.*

4. *Judge no one. Everyone is dealing with something, and we try to hide it from the world. The people who allow themselves to be seen and are honest are the ones worth your time.*

5. *Take self-responsibility. If you're unhappy it's inside your brain, work on you and focus on what you can control.*

6. *Nobody can fix you until you choose to fix yourself first and find your 'WHY' to live your life and get well.*

7. *Every day is a new day. If you make a mistake with others, apologise fast. Letting a hurt heart bleed too long is just not worth it.*

8. *If you feel like the world is going to end, go to bed early and sleep. There is hope in a new dawn.*

9. *What you eat and drink directly impacts your mood and energy – food is mood.*

10. *Exercise, sleep, good nutrition, faith and love are the best specialists you will ever need to make you well. Don't underestimate your own intelligence to use these things to empower you.*

11. *Don't give your power away to other people. Care about yourself and your health – you are worth it. You may have to do the work to find the key to your door, but it's worth it.*

12. *Nobody else lives in your body, or lives your life, so take all advice with a grain of salt.*

13. *Let people, things and situations that don't make you happy go.*

14. *Visualise the new life you want. Don't pine for the past, rebuild a new life day by day.*

15. *Practice gratitude daily for the small things.*

There are two moments for opportunity, the present and tomorrow. Yesterday is gone and you can't get it back. But you can build a new tomorrow out of the mud. I'm okay, you're okay.

Growth happens in the dirt.

Katie x

Resources

1. The concussion traffic light system
2. 'What helps/what hurts?'
3. Specialist entry: Physiotherapy for concussion by Colin Hancock
4. Specialist entry: Occupational Therapy by Vicki Gould
5. Specialist entry: Strategies from the Amen Clinics
6. The Glycaemic Load for concussion
7. Specialist entry: EMDR by Mark Grant
8. Specialist entry: Neuro optometry by Brenton Clark
9. Specialist entry: Alternative eye therapies for concussion by Bradley Pillay (Neuro Optometrist)
10. Self-help eye exercises by Ryan O'Connor

The concussion traffic light system

The traffic light system for concussion triggers is a way to stay focussed on how you are feeling at any one time. During the recovery process, you may shift from orange to red very quickly. If you understand what your 'orange' state is, you can quickly take a brain bath to avoid slipping into 'red'. Use this method to communicate to your loved ones what 'colour' you are in on any one day. This will aid them to support you if they notice you are starting to 'orange out' and recommend that you take a brain bath. Understanding the traffic light system (and you may have individual orange and red responses that differ from these) will teach you how to care for yourself before hitting the 'red' stage. For example:

Mila woke feeling well, but after a few hours she started to develop a headache (orange). Her mother noticed that she was squinting with her eyes and starting to get irritable (orange). Because they had to run errands, Mila didn't take a brain bath, and while they were at the supermarket she started to cry (red) and experience major anxiety (red). In the car on the way home, Mila started screaming at her mother, 'You don't understand me, I want to kill myself.' (red). If Mila had been able to brain bath at orange, things would not escalate.

know your 'concussion lights'

Green

Feeling calm
Slept well
Taking regular brain baths
Minimizing screens
Can think clearly
Good nutrition
Planning and pacing
Exercising
Can cope with noise and light
Conversation is ok
Pain low

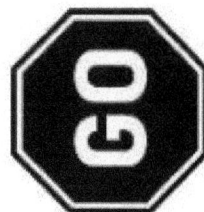

Orange

Noise and light is starting to irritate - sensory issues
Mixing up words
Feeling tired
Pain starting
Eyes may feel tired
Conversation is a struggle
Small things are irritating
Thoughts are jumbled
Memory is struggling
Mood dropping

TAKE A BRAIN BATH NOW

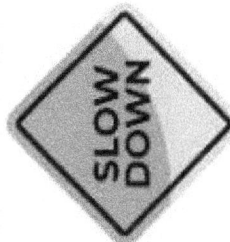

Red

Extreme pain
Crying
Rage attack
Extreme sensitivity to noise and stimulus
Fighting with loved ones
Stuck on thoughts
Extreme fatigue
Memory bad
Migraine
Extreme mood swings

DESENSITISE IMMEDIATELY

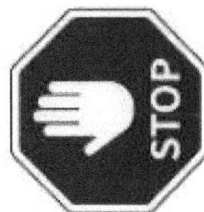

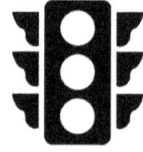

What are your 'concussion lights'?

Mark down the feelings, behaviours and symptoms in each column. Know what your triggers are, what helps, what hurts, and notice the orange column. This will help you to know when to take a brain break. When you 'green' you are feeling well. When you are 'orange' you are starting to be symptomatic. When you are red, you are feeling very symptomatic.

GREEN	ORANGE	RED

What helps? What hurts?

Make a list of the things that really help you below.

The things that when you do them you feel better, and when you don't do them, you feel worse. It may be making sure you exercise or eat breakfast. List everything that helps so you can see what works for you. Then in the other column, write down everything that hurts your brain (or when you do them you feel worse). This will help to get clarity and create a toolbox for your recovery to implement or avoid daily.

WHAT HELPS	WHAT HURTS

'Physiotherapy for concussion'

Specialist entry: by Colin Hancock concussion physiotherapist

Katie: How Colin Hancock changed my life.
Before my initial appointment with Colin, I knew NOTHING
about concussion or its effects on the brain. Colin's experience
as a physiotherapist working with concussion in sport was the
key to unlocking symptoms that I thought were just me being
'crazy'. Finding a physiotherapist who has knowledge of
concussion rehabilitation is key to helping you start to heal
your body.

My name is Colin Hancock, a New Zealand and Australia-
registered physiotherapist with 27 years' experience. My
original interest in concussion injury stemmed from my own
concussion injuries playing rugby in the 1980s and 90s. Back
then very little was done to manage this injury and often
sportspeople simply returned to play the following week, with
inadequate recovery. Eventually I stopped playing contact sport
due to the progressive ease to which I was getting this injury
with less force.

My professional background in treating concussion injury
started 12 years ago when I attended a physiotherapy course in

managing sports injuries sideline. Part of the course reflected on recognising concussion, the initial management (usually just physical and cognitive rest back then), then how to return people back to sport when it was judged they had recovered. The science behind how to manage concussion has advanced dramatically since then.

Concussion hacks:

What should a person with concussion do immediately after a concussion injury?

1. After recognition that a concussion injury has likely occurred, immediate removal from the risk of collisions and falls should occur. Recent research has given us astounding knowledge. It's shown that playing on for a further 15 minutes will extend recovery time by approximately 30 days.

2. A neck sprain injury very commonly occurs alongside concussion injury. In fact, it's often very difficult to discern whether the cause of symptoms comes from a neck sprain or concussion injury as symptoms are similar (headache, dizziness, foggy head, nausea, fatigue). Ruling out a more serious neck injury is important. If there are pins and needles, numbness or muscle weakness in your arms or legs, or central neck pain with limited ability to

turn your neck (less the 30 degrees either way) it is critical you seek medical attention and get an x-ray.

3. If you can rule out a significant neck injury, having 48hrs of complete physical and cognitive (thinking) rest has been shown to reduce the brain's need for energy, allowing it to recover quickly. Over-exerting yourself by thinking too much or being too physically active in the first two days has been shown to slow recovery. This means limiting driving, no drinking, keeping off your phone or computer, and keeping things quiet and relaxed.

4. After 48hrs, research shows adding low key physical activity below where symptoms feel worse helps the brain recover. Often this is just going for a walk for 30mins a day with sunglasses on (to limit brightness) in a quiet place with not too much complexity to look at such as at a marketplace or sportsground with lots of people around.

5. The eyes use up near to 50% of the brain's energy to function. After concussion the eyes can get stuck in a strained focus position and unable to relax. Limiting the effort of the eyes can make someone with concussion feel much less fatigued.

One eye relaxation technique is "Eye cupping" for brief periods. This can allow the eyes to relax.

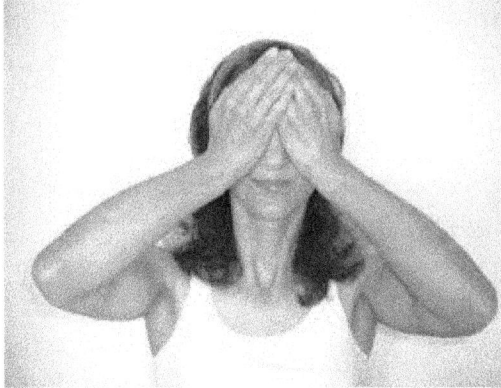

A trick that is often used to reduce the demand on the brain is placing a small strip of cloudy Sellotape on the inner 1cm of the sunglasses (nearest the nose) on each side. This reduces the demand on the brain by stopping the need for the brain to calculate 3D vision. This effectively creates a situation where the right eye looks at the right side of the body, and the left eye looks at the left side. This can often make brain fatigue reduce dramatically.

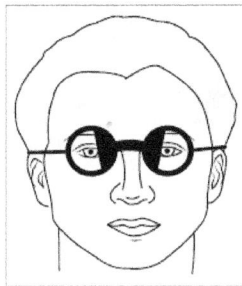

Picture sourced from Amplify Eye Care

6. A neck sprain can be the source of significant concussion-like symptoms and ideally getting help from someone skilled in recovering neck mobility and control such as a physiotherapist, osteopath or chiropractor often helps. If these are not available to you there are certain things that you can do yourself to ease neck related symptoms.

7. Ensure you maintain a reasonable posture. The more slouched you are the more the neck muscles must work.

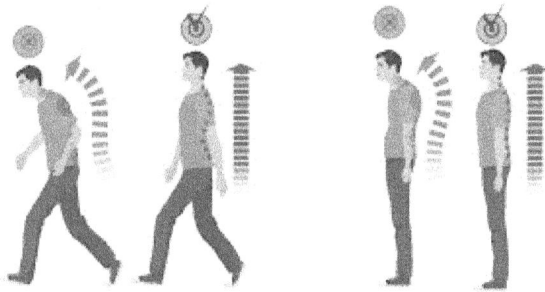

Picture from Ergo Impact

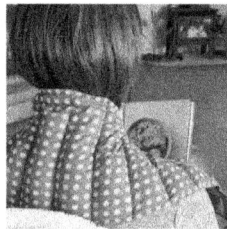

Applying a warm wheat bag /hot water bottle to the neck muscles can relax the muscles a little, easing the headache.

8. Certain stretches are known to help stretch the high neck muscles at the base of the skull which are most often tight after a neck sprain. One particularly useful stretch is to tuck your chin in, then downward pressure on top of your head. This stretches the muscle just under the skull and upper few neck bones which commonly cause headaches. Hold the stretch for 15-20 seconds for 2-3 times.

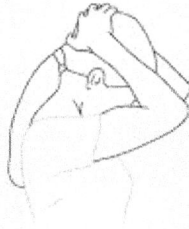

Picture from Healthline

9. Recovering rotation of the neck when the neck is less painful is also important. Use a chin tuck and then rotation, keeping to within the discomfort, but not painful, zone usually slowly recovers range of movement over days.

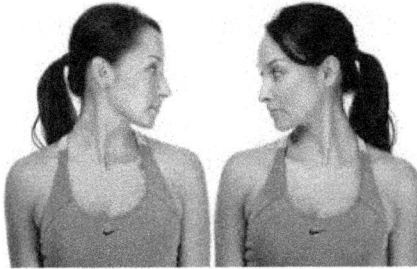

What can be done about sleep?

Often those with concussion have a frustratingly dysfunctional sleep pattern. Either they can't get to sleep or get to sleep but wake up too early and can't get back to sleep or sleep too much. Below are some tricks to restore sleep to normal again.

During the day:

- Avoid naps for longer than one hour during the day as this can impact your sleep at night. You may be better having a meditation break versus a deep sleep during the day.
- Try to keep physically active through the day, rather than before bed.
- Follow the directions of your prescribed medication correctly. If you are unsure about which of your medications will help you sleep better, discuss this with your doctor or pharmacist.

In the evening:

- Replace stimulant drinks with warm drinks that don't contain caffeine.
- Avoid entirely or limit the amount of alcohol and only drink with dinner.

- Avoid activities that get the brain hyped up before bedtime.
- Plan to do relaxing, pleasant tasks in the hour before bed (e.g. listening to relaxing music)
- Try to establish a regular routine and get ready to go to bed at about the same time every night.
- Try to get up about the same time each day, regardless of how you feel.
- If you are off work, get up and go to bed at the same time as you would have when you were working.
- Avoid bright lights and devices with bright screens as they can suppress the sleep hormone melatonin. Use a night mode filter on your phone/laptop if you are using them.
- Use dim red-tinted lights in the evening for a few hours before you sleep.

During the night:

- Deal with worries before bed or write them down to address tomorrow.
- Use relaxation techniques and mental distractions. Relaxation / Breathing / Distraction / Stopping unhelpful thoughts. You may need to repeat these several times but try to stay calm.

- If you can't sleep, get up and do something peaceful until you feel ready to sleep again, then return to bed.
- Remember, if you are relaxing you are still getting rest
- Keep sleep spaces dark.
- Try to avoid using sleep spaces for work activities like studying / schoolwork.

How do I get back to work, school and sport?

When symptoms have reduced to low enough levels at rest, a gradual return to either work or school is recommended. This can start to occur even within the first week after injury if symptoms have subsided. If symptoms increase on return to learning or work, it may be a sign that the level of work or learning is still too much for the brain energy levels at that time and a slightly lower level of learning or work is needed. This may mean limited hours or school/ work or the need for multiple brain breaks throughout the work or school day are required.

Return-to-learn (RTL) strategy

TABLE 1.

Return-to-Learn Plan

Stage	Activity	Objective
No activity	Complete cognitive rest — no school, no homework, no reading, no texting, no video games, no computer work.	Recovery
Gradual reintroduction of cognitive activity	Relax previous restrictions on activities and add back for short periods of time (5-15 minutes at a time).	Gradual controlled increase in subsymptom threshold cognitive activities.
Homework at home before school work at school	Homework in longer increments (20-30 minutes at a time).	Increase cognitive stamina by repetition of short periods of self-paced cognitive activity.
School re-entry	Part day of school after tolerating 1-2 cumulative hours of homework at home.	Re-entry into school with accommodations to permit controlled subsymptom threshold increase in cognitive load.
Gradual reintegration into school	Increase to full day of school.	Accommodations decrease as cognitive stamina improves.
Resumption of full cognitive workload	Introduce testing, catch up with essential work.	Full return to school; may commence Return-to-Play protocol (see Step 2 in Table 2).

Source: Master CL, Gioia GA, Leddy JJ, Grady MF

Taken from Semantic Scholar

Balance training:

Balance can commonly be affected after concussion. Doing balancing exercises will improve this over time. Here are some useful balance tasks to try.

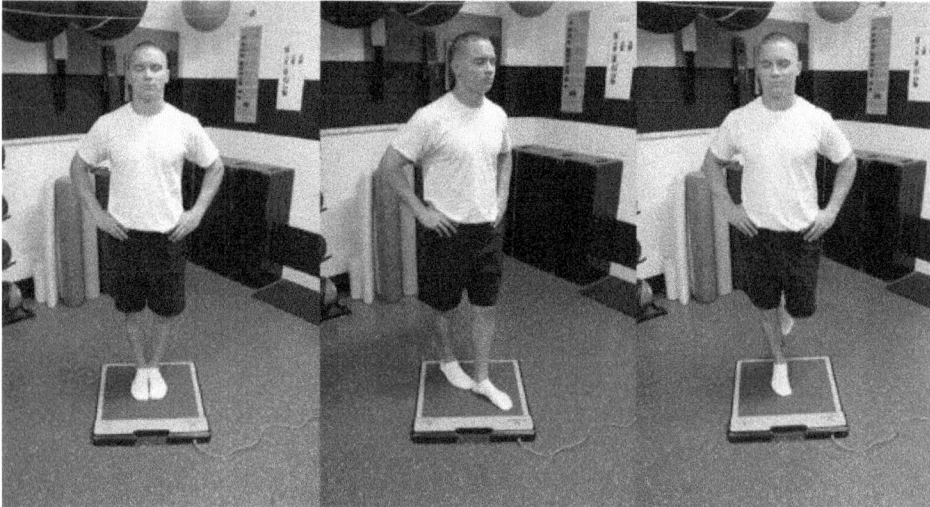

Use the corner of the room with a chair in front to make sure you're safe from falling too far should you lose your balance.

Start with feet together in the first positional challenge.

1. eyes open balance
2. eyes open move eyes side to side, up down
3. eyes open move head side to side or up and down
4. eyes closed
5. eyes closed move head side to side or up and down

Progressions: aim 30secs in each position before you progress through progressions. Most people can only cope with doing these exercises for about 5minutes at a time, but they can be done 3 times a day.

To advance to a harder position try stride stance – follow progressions as for above. Then finally if able try single leg balance – progressions as above.

Vertigo treatment

Some people with concussion experience vertigo (often referred to as BPPV), where you feel like the room spins when you move from position to position or turn your head too fast. Treatment for this is quite effective and sometimes gives almost immediate relief, however ensuring the right corrective exercises requires assessment by someone skilled in understanding vertigo and knowing what specific head movement will ease the problem.

If you are living in a place where no health professionals are available who know how to treat vertigo, it may be worth trying the most common treatment strategy for easing vertigo (in around 80% of cases).

Firstly, perform a test called the Dix Hallpike test on the right and left: see YouTube link below.

https://www. youtube. com/watch?v=D6qEdlFVxig

As there is no therapist to assess your eye movement when you get vertigo, you'll need to discern which side (left or right Dix Hallpike) gave the most vertigo. This is the side you should try the Epley repositioning technique on (see YouTube video).

If this fails to ease the vertigo it may be that your vertigo is more complex, and I'd recommend seeking a review by a health professional adept at managing vertigo. This is commonly a physiotherapist, GP, osteopath or neurologist.

How to return to sport?

After you have successfully returned to school or work, the next challenge is to return to recreational activity. This may also be activities that involve further risk of falls or collisions. Ensuring you have fully recovered before returning to these risky activities is very important as the brain is vulnerable to even more injury when it is still healing from the first concussion. The process most people follow is laid out below in a step-by-step process (by pleasantonrage.com):

RAGE Concussion Return-to-Play Protocol

DATE	STAGE	ACTIVITY	EXAMPLE	GOAL
	1	Rest	• Short walks encouraged	Recovery and reduction of symptoms
WRITTEN PHYSICAL CLEARANCE REQUIRED "BEGIN RTP PROTOCOL"				
	2	Light aerobic activity	• 10-15 minutes of brisk walk/stationary bike	Increase heart rate
	3	Moderate aerobic activity	• Easy jogging • Body weight resistance exercise	Increase heart rate Increase forces on brain
	4	Sport specific exercise	• Full speed running • Ball handling (juggling, passing, dribbling) • No heading	Add total body movement Increase heart rate
	5	Non-contact training	• Multiple player drills (rondo, flying chases) • Agility and conditioning • No scrimmage • No heading	Increase acceleration, deceleration and rotational forces
WRITTEN PHYSICIAN CLEARANCE REQUIRED "CLEARED FOR CONTACT"				
	6	Full-contact training	• Normal, unrestricted training	Restore confidence, assess readiness to play

250

Occupational Therapy

Specialist entry by: Vicki Gould, Occupational Therapist
(OTNZR)

Katie: How Vicki Gould changed my life.
When I was referred to the concussion team, Vicki Gould was
my first specialist. She made me realise that everything I was
experiencing were normal effects of post-concussion syndrome.
The practical steps that she suggested helped me to navigate
the journey of recovery and know that change is hard and that
consistency amidst failure can bring about massive changes.

As an occupational therapist (OT) working with clients with
concussion for many years, I have learnt everyone's
presentation is different. However, there are themes that arise,
and the literature tells us the following:

There are 3 types of concussion – *mild, moderate* and *severe.*

All can have an impact on functioning in the days and weeks
following. A small percentage of clients can have symptoms for
longer.

There are 5 subtypes of concussion. And a mixture of these symptoms is why concussion recovery usually requires an interdisciplinary approach to rehabilitation. These are:

- Cognitive – brain functioning for things like memory, concentration, thinking speed.
- Ocular-motor – problems with the visual system affecting performance.
- Headaches.
- Vestibular – Disruption to the central vestibular system (nerves and structures in the inner ear) that involves movement and orientation of the head and body to space.
- Mood – changes in mood and possibly anxiety.

We also know that people can have concussion-related sleep disturbance and cervical strain associated with the injury. When I first meet a client, I complete an initial concussion assessment and in doing that decide what other health professionals needed to be involved.

Depending on need, this may be a neuro physiotherapist, a musculoskeletal (MSK) physiotherapist for a neck assessment and treatment, a psychologist and occupational therapy. We can also utilise a speech language therapist and a nurse if needed. Neuro-optometry can be invaluable depending on need.

So, what is covered when you work with an Occupational Therapist for concussion?

Education and advice about:

1. **What is concussion?**

   It is a mild traumatic brain injury. *It may occur without the loss of consciousness*, in fact most people do not lose consciousness. It can cause temporary chemical changes to the brain cells which may result in short-lived impairment to neurological function.

2. **Expectations for recovery**

   Most people fully recover from a concussion within a few weeks, some even a few days. Some may take a few months and a small minority may have to manage symptoms longer than a few months. Be reassured though, if you are very symptomatic, *you will improve.* Tackle the issues methodically and get support. The literature varies about this, but I think a referral sooner rather than later to a concussion service generates the best outcomes.

3. **Energy/ Fatigue**

   It wasn't that long ago that people with a concussion were told to go to bed and rest, sleep it off, or do nothing or a while. Those days have passed. With a severe concussion it may be necessary to rest most of the first 2 or 3 days but now we ask people to intermingle rest with activity. Complete resting for too long can lead to deconditioning and a prolonged recovery. So now, depending on your energy/fatigue levels, we suggest you move between activity, rest, activity, etc. How you do this depends on how you are feeling, of course. An example may be 60 minutes of activity, 5 minutes rest or 30 minutes activity, 2 to 3 minutes rest, with a short sleep in the afternoon of 30 to 60 minutes. *It is vital any daytime sleeping does not interfere with your night sleep so keep an eye on that.*

I worked with a client who needed to rest 15 minutes, be active 15 minutes and so on. We increased the activity timeframe by a few minutes each day and reduced the rest period by a few minutes each day. He eventually got to a stage of being able to function normally. The 60 minute / 5-minute scenario often helps most people.

Some people have difficulty identifying when they are tired until they are so fatigued they can barely function. Try and catch your tiredness before it is exhaustion and have a rest sooner rather than later. You may need to ask people you are close to, to help you identify your signs.

Irritability, slowed thinking and headaches can give you a clue. Don't ignore and push through these symptoms. You may have to function with a headache or when you are under par, but learn about the variations of these symptoms and a blanket ignoring of them won't resolve the issues.

For the rest time, we call it a zero-stimulation break. No noise (ear plugs can be useful, turn off all background noise), no light (eye masks are useful) and quieten thinking. Think of puffy clouds moving slowly in the blue sky or gentle waves breaking on the beach. For a few people, a 5-minute recording of calming sounds may be needed but this is not the ideal as your brain is activated through listening. The purpose of this zero-stimulation break is to allow the brain and nervous system to calm down and reduce overwhelm to the brain. If you are out and about, you may find doing this in the car helpful. For example, just before you go into the supermarket, sit in the car and rest for a few minutes, cover your eyes with your hands and calm your breathing.

For the time of activity, if possible, I suggest you rotate between a cognitive task (such as reading a magazine or a simple crossword) then a physical task (such as walking), then a housework or food prep task (such as vacuuming or preparing food standing at the bench) Mindful activities are also good, such as knitting, gardening, a small mechanical job in your shed or a jigsaw puzzle. What you do will depend on your interests and your symptoms.

Depending on how they make you feel, screens may be okay but in my experience many people cannot cope with screens for more than 10 to 20 minutes at one time shortly after a concussion and you want to avoid getting sore eyes or a headache by screen over use. If screens are important to you (as with most people these days) try building up screen use by a few minutes a day. They may need to be alongside visual rehab.

4. **Pace your activity!**
   Approach your day in a calm, methodical manner, being grateful for what you can achieve at this time. *Do you need to lower your expectations?* Be kind to your brain, *give yourself permission to recover*. If an afternoon sleep is required, I suggest you set an alarm and see if 60 minutes is long enough to get you through the rest of the

afternoon and evening. As you improve, reduce this nap until you no longer need it.

5. **Sleep**

Unfortunately, an injury to your brain can disrupt your sleep patterns and this is often the last thing you need if daytime fatigue is an issue. In my experience, following a concussion, this will improve so don't stress about it; try and go with the flow and put in good strategies. My top tips for improving your sleep are:

- No matter the weather, get at least 10 to 30 minutes of morning light, outside, *within the first 30 minutes of waking up*. Take a cup of tea into the garden or go for a walk (if your balance is OK). This helps to set or re-set your circadian rhythm (24-hour body clock) so by the time you hit the sack at night, your body knows it is time to sleep. Thanks to this top tip, my dog gets 2 walks a day and this helps me to fall asleep at night.
- Don't over-rest during the day but avoid getting so over-tired that your brain feels wired at the end of the day. Like an over-tired baby, it is possible to get scratchy and restless without sufficient brain breaks.

- Avoid caffeine and food for a few hours prior to bedtime. Exactly how long varies per person but I avoid all caffeine from after lunch.
- Good bedtime routines – same habits and time frames.
- Google breathing exercises for sleep.
- No screens 30 to 60 minutes before bed.
- If you can't get to sleep, after 20 or so minutes, get up, maybe have a warm drink and read a boring magazine for half an hour then return to bed and try again. Repeat if necessary. I don't think lying in bed tossing and turning for ages helps.
- You may find that prior to your concussion, you didn't have to worry about such things, but because your brain is in recovery different strategies may be needed.

6. **Brain stuff: Attention, concentration, information processing and memory**

Brain fog, trouble finding the right word, losing your train of thought or just having trouble thinking normally, difficulty reading and blocking out distractions, can all be scary. And I am sure there is often concern that these symptoms will continue. These are common symptoms of a concussion and are transient. *Horrible – yes, permanent – no.* Have you noticed you are better in the morning than the afternoon? This is because the brain gets overloaded as the day goes on and it is telling you it can't cope! I consider good energy management helps the brain more than anything else (see above). Also, strategies like turning off background noise; turning down the phone volume; make yourself written lists so you are not relying on your memory; lower your expectations of what your brain can cope with; plan and pace activities over your day and week; repeat information back to people; use diaries or calendars.

Coping with a busy household can be hard work. Start by being kind to yourself. What housework chores can wait? Simplify the meals. So the kids might have more screen time than usual – it is not forever. Call on friends or family. Would you help them if the boot was on the other foot? GIVE YOURSELF PERMISSION TO REHABILITATE AND RECOVER!

7. **Visual issues**

   The OT or physio can assess your vision and provide exercises to improve things or decide to refer you to a neuro optometrist. The main thing for you to decide is about screens. Are they affecting you and how much and how? Sore eyes? Headaches? If yes, limit screens of any type to below symptom level until you get some advice and rehab.

8. **Discussion about driving**

   If in doubt, leave it out. Please do not drive if you are fatigued, dizzy, have distracting pain or visual issues, or for any other reason you have that will affect your driving. If transport is an issue for you and you know you are not up to driving, seek a support network to help you.

As you improve, build up your return to driving cautiously. If possible, trial being a passenger first. If you are fine with that, plan a short trip. Ideally your GP or concussion therapist should give you the OK to return to driving after severe symptoms.

Strategies from the Amen Clinics

Authorised excerpt from Amen University. For more information read The Brain Warrior's Way *by Daniel Amen and Tana Amen. Practitioners and those interested in studying more about brain health can visit* https://www.amenuniversity.com *What follows has been authorised by the Amen Clinics.*

The Amen Clinics have identified three key strategies to help your brain function:

1. Brain envy
2. Avoid anything that hurts the brain
3. Engage in regular brain healthy habits

Dr Amen writes: 'Mild traumatic brain injuries are a major cause of psychiatric illness, and many mental health professionals miss it in patients because they rarely look at the brains of their patients. Brain injuries are a major cause of drug and alcohol abuse, depression, anxiety, ADHD symptoms, suicide and homelessness. You are not stuck with the brain you have. You can make it better by using the program outlined in this book (*The Brain Warrior's Way*).'

Dr Amen has a free brain type test available online at https://www.brainhealthassessment.com/ in which you can see what your brain needs to function at its best. Knowing your brain symptoms during concussion can help you tailor your nutritional pathway to heal. There are five primary brain types (and 11 blended types)

1. Balanced (no issues – not concussion people ☺). This type suits a well-balanced low glycaemic index diet.
2. Spontaneous (ADHD type, creative, out of the box thinker, restless, easily distracted, focussed only when interested). Dr Amen has shown this type does better on a high protein low carbohydrate diet to increase *dopamine* with high intensity exercise.
3. Persistent (strong willed, gets stuck on thoughts, holds on to hurts, notices fault in self and others). Dr Amen has shown this type does better on a *serotonin* boosting diet. Include sweet potato, quinoa and legumes and physical exercise.
4. Sensitive (feels deeply, empathic, pessimistic, negative thoughts). Dr Amen has shown more omega 3 foods, vitamin D and exercise can help this type and a balanced low glycaemic index diet.

5. Cautious (prepared, motivated, reserved, busy minded, restless). Dr Amen has shown this type needs more magnesium, vitamin B6 and *GABA* foods, and exercise with a balanced low glycaemic index diet.

Foods that make you smarter and happier

Serotonin is the 'don't worry be happy' neurotransmitter. Responsible for mood stability, sleep regulation, appetite control and social engagement. People who are low in serotonin crave carbohydrate-rich foods such as pasta, bread and chocolate. Complex carbohydrates from plant foods can help:

Sweet potatoes, hummus, apples, pears, peaches, blueberries, bananas, oranges, grapes, figs, mangoes, pineapple.

Dopamine is the neurotransmitter associated with motivation, relevance, focus and the ability to experience pleasure. Low dopamine is associated with ADD, lack of focus and lower motivation. Protein foods can help:

Seafood, poultry, lean meat, lima beans and lentils, nuts, pumpkin and sesame seeds, protein powders (low sugar) and high protein vegetables like broccoli and spinach. Also add green tea.

Acetylcholine is the neurotransmitter for learning, memory and association. This is especially important for traumatic head injuries. Foods that have this are: eggs, liver, lecithin, salmon and shrimp.

GABA is an inhibitory neurotransmitter which calms, stabilises and grounds. Decreased GABA leads to anxiety, irritability and some cyclic mood disorders. Foods rich in GABA are: broccoli, nuts and lentils.

Important nutrition principles from the Amen Clinic

1. The brain consumes 20-30 per cent of the calories you consume. By focussing on eating low glycaemic load health foods you feed your brain and body.
2. Always eat breakfast focussing on eating healthy proteins in the morning to wake up the brain.
3. Eat complex carbohydrates at night to help with relaxation and sleep.
4. Balance your blood sugars to help stabilise energy and mood. Focus on combining low 'sugar' sources of fat, protein and carbohydrate at every meal.

5. Your brain is 60 per cent fat (solid weight). Include in your diet fatty fish, nuts and seeds, avocado, omega 3 supplements and oils such as coconut, olive oil, macadamia and ghee.
6. Avoid processed food and artificial sweeteners.
7. Use brain-boosting herbs and spices in your cooking.
8. Drink at least ½ your body weight in ounces of water daily (if you are very overweight contact a practitioner about correct amounts). Reduce or eliminate completely alcohol and caffeine.
9. Load your plate with a rainbow of vegetables and fruits for nutrients and antioxidants. Experts suggest eating 25-35g of fibre daily to balance blood sugars, feel full and help with healthy bowels.

The Glycaemic Load for concussion

The glycaemic load (GL) of food is a number that estimates how much the food will raise a person's blood glucose level after it is eaten. One unit of glycaemic load approximates the effect of eating one gram of glucose.

Stabilising your blood sugar so that you get a constant flow of energy from your food is key.

If we view nutrition like how we drive a car, some foods will cause a massive stop in your concussion recovery (red foods), some will slow you down (orange) and others will allow you to 'go' (green).

The traffic light system shows you what foods to go with, slow down on and stop. Foods high in fibre will slow blood sugars – so for all carbohydrates, aim to eat high fibre.

If you are eating 'red' foods, combine with a protein and fat source to help slow the insulin spike.

GREEN FOODS HAVE LOW IMPACT ON BLOOD SUGARS - GREEN FOR GO!

Animal foods: chicken, beef, lamb, turkey, bison, fish, shrimp, shellfish, eggs, gelatin (no sugar)

Vegetables: Alfalfa, artichokes, asparagus, bamboo shoots, bean sprouts, bok choy, broccoli, brussels sprouts, cabbage carrots, cauliflower, celery, chard/silver beet, collard/mustard greens, cucumbers, green beans, kale, leeks, lettuces, mushrooms, okra, olives, onions, peppers, radishes, snow peas, spinach, summer squash, turnips, water chestnuts, zucchini

Fruits (limit to two servings daily): Apples, apricots, avocado, berries, cherries, grapes, grapefruit, kiwifruit, lemons, limes, nectarines, oranges, peaches, pears, plums, tangerines, tomatoes

Legumes: Beans (all kinds except canned baked beans), black eyed peas, chickpeas, hummus, lentils, peanuts, split peas, pea protein powder (low sugar)

Nuts/Seeds: Almonds, Brazil, cashews, hazelnuts, nut butters (no added sugar), pecans, pistachios, walnuts, chia, pumpkin, sesame, sunflower, flaxseed

Dairy: Cheese, yoghurt (no added sugar), whey protein powder (low sugar)

Grain alternatives: Konjac noodles, high fibre legume pastas, low carb bread and wraps

Fats are low GL: opt for olive oil, coconut oil, ghee, butter, macadamia oil, avocado oil

Desserts & sweet treats: Dark chocolate (70% and above, dairy & sugar free)

Sweeteners: Fructose (but goes to the liver – avoid), agave (goes to the liver – avoid), erythritol, stevia, xylitol

ORANGE FOODS HAVE MORE IMPACT ON BLOOD SUGARS – ORANGE FOR SLOW!

Animal foods: Meat products with added wheat in a crumb or added ingredients

Vegetables (leaving the skin on can increase fibre and reduce GL load): Acorn squash, beets, butternut squash, green peas, parsnips, pumpkin, sweet potatoes, yams, potatoes

Fruits: Bananas, cantaloupe, honeydew, mango, papaya, pineapple, watermelon

Legumes: Peanut butter, sugar sweetened

Nuts/Seeds: any type of nut/seed with added sugar or honey, baked beans

Dairy: Milk

Grains: Amaranth, barley, bread (stone ground, sprouted grain, high fibre), breakfast cereal (high fibre), brown rice, buckwheat, corn, farro, steel cut oats, quinoa, rye, wheat berries, wild rice

Desserts & sweet treats: Ice cream, milk chocolate

Sweeteners: Honey, table sugar

RED FOODS HAVE A MASSIVE IMPACT ON BLOOD SUGARS – RED FOR CHOOSE A GREEN ALTERNATIVE.

Vegetables: Boiled potatoes, fries, potato chips

Fruits: Dates, dried fruit, fruit juices and drinks, raisins

Legumes: Candy or chocolate/yoghurt coated peanuts

Nuts or seeds: covered in chocolate or candy

Dairy: Flavoured and sweetened milk/yoghurt/ice-cream

Grains: Bread including bagels, buns, corn bread, muffins, pitas, rolls, most white and wheat breads (low fibre), low fibre breakfast cereals, couscous, crackers, pancakes, pasta, pizza, popcorn, pretzels, rice cakes, stuffing, taco shells, tortilla, waffle, white rice, granola bars

Desserts & sweet treats: Brownies, cake, candy, chips, cookies, custards, doughnuts, fruit roll ups, pies, sorbet, muesli/granola bars

Sweeteners: glucose

Sneaky sugars: Tomato, barbeque, sweet chilli sauce, anything touted LOW FAT, date health bars and muesli bars, jams and breakfast spreads, instant oats, instant sachet coffees/hot chocolate, low fibre bread and crackers.

EMDR (Eye movement desensitization and reprocessing)

Specialist entry: by Mark Grant MA

Katie: How Mark Grant changed my life:
When I read Mark's book Change Your Brain, Change Your Pain
I wasn't happy. To read that most of the pain actually occurs in
our brains and not in our bodies left me in disbelief. But as I
started to implement EMDR as part of my daily routine
(listening to the Mark Grant EMDR audio tracks), my
relationship with pain changed and I felt I had more control of
my symptoms.

I (Mark Grant) was looking for more effective ways to treat chronic pain and medically unexplained symptoms in the early 1990s when I heard about Eye Movement Desensitization and Reprocessing (EMDR). It sounded unlike anything I had ever come across and it felt attractive to a lover of the new and novel (but not too 'fringy') ideas.

EMDR is based on the Adaptive Information Processing (AIP) Model which posits that all human beings have an innate capacity to process experience in an adaptive way. Every experience is or should be an opportunity to learn something useful for the future.

The details of AIP include the human sensory system (our 5 senses), the brain (particularly its reward and danger systems) and the various organs of our body responsible for maintenance of physical health. The danger system, or flight-fight response, alerts us to threat, and then other parts of the brain learn whatever lessons need to be learned, and that experience gets filed away as a memory. But with traumatic events, the extreme intensity of the feelings inhibits the brain's ability to process our responses to the event, leading to its constantly being replayed (i.e., PTSD - intrusive thoughts, irrational anxiety, avoidance).

PTSD also involves a kind of dissociation between mental and physical experience; at one level we know we survived and whatever happened is in the past, but at another deeper level it still feels very much in the present and/or like it could happen again at any moment. In reliving the event we may also re-experience any physical or emotional pain that occurred at the time, or delayed pain due to biochemical imbalances associated with chronic PTSD (decreased cortisol, increased inflammation). The 'memory' is therefore more than what happened and its immediate affective legacy; it is also long-term psycho-physiological effects such as fatigue, cortisol imbalances, nociplastic changes and impaired immune functioning which may or not be related to a discrete injury or illness but are always in excess of normal pain. As pain expert Ronald Melzack once said:

'Stressors have destructive effects on muscle, skeletal and neural tissue, which may become the immediate basis of pain or a provider basis for the devastating effects of later mild injuries in which the severity of pain is disproportionately far greater and will be expected from the injury.'

At its heart the EMDR method relied on a dual focus of attention process wherein the patient recalls the distressing memory associated with their current problems (including feelings, images, thoughts) and simultaneously pays attention to external alternating visual, auditory or tactile) stimuli.

Because the first stimuli were visual, the name EMDR centred on eye movements. Before learning EMDR I witnessed a colleague demonstrate the method with a PTSD sufferer in which symptoms (anxiety, panic attacks) that this person had struggled with for years after a serious car accident literally faded away as she focused on her therapist's hand moving backwards and forwards at eye level. I could see the tension literally draining out of her body. After the EMDR clients were able to talk about the accident calmly, as though it was just something that happened. Such a profound transformation in such a short time seemed miraculous, but also proof of the AIP model. I was also struck by the decrease in physiological symptoms, the calmness, the mental detachment the patient reported.

In those days exposure was a very popular treatment – but it could take weeks and often involved great distress for the patient. They were often left with persistent symptoms which meant they constantly had to practise anxiety-management techniques such as breathing to contain. The result was that they still had to live with 'it' to some degree. EMDR seemed to be able to facilitate resolution of problems much more completely, more easily and more quickly, without the need to keep practising anxiety management strategies.

One of my earliest cases involved a grandmother who came to me complaining of jaw pain (she had not been able to eat solid food for a year) following the traumatic death of her grandson due to medical misadventure. Maria wept inconsolably as she recounted these events, describing the loss as a 'tragedy' and 'destruction of life.' She was otherwise healthy and generally resilient having coped with many other life stressors well.

Following the usual preliminaries (history, assessment, preparation) I instructed Maria to focus on the memory of the death, the pain in her jaw and her heart, and her negative thoughts ('I'm helpless') while she focused on bilateral stimulation. Almost immediately she reported the pain her heart felt 'lighter', and she started making opening and closing movements with her mouth and touching her jaw. This continued for a few more minutes of bilateral stimulation where the grief and pain visibly drained from Maria's face. After perhaps 5 minutes, Maria was extending her jaw fully, slightly disbelievingly.

When I asked how she felt now she reported she felt calm. When I asked her about the memory of her grandson's death, she reported feeling free of all pain and sadness and could now remember her grandson 'with love, not pain'. She left the office declaring that she was going home to enjoy a nice piece of steak.

Maria's story illustrates a relatively simple example of trauma-related pain or somatic symptom disorder as its now known (formerly 'conversion disorder' or hysteria). More commonly, medically unexplained pain involves a combination of capital 'T' trauma and small 't' trauma such as emotional neglect, family violence and other forms of adversity.

In such cases, which is most of my patients, EMDR must be integrated with other strategies such as hypnosis, ego-state work and somatic-focused psychotherapy. Individuals with complex trauma histories are often exhausted and have a very low opinion of themselves, meaning their nervous systems lack the resources to respond to EMDR alone.

For example, a nurse sought my help for chronic pain after injuring her back whilst lifting a patient. By the time she came to see me, Stacey had been in pain for 8 years. She was taking handfuls of painkillers to get through the day, and she was tired and depressed. She had recurring thoughts of killing herself. She had not worked for the last two years; her marriage was on the verge of collapse and the couple had had to sell the family home because of financial problems. Unfortunately, like many chronic pain sufferers, prior to her back injury Stacey had also endured much adversity ranging from childhood emotional neglect to a botched pelvic mesh surgery. Stacey was thus affected by a raft of problems, including attachment trauma, migration, school bullying, work stress, a botched medical procedure and her injury and pain. Underneath it all Stacey had a very low opinion of herself and a very limited ability to ask for what she needed in life. EMDR alone could not undo the chronic pain that Stacey was experiencing – her nervous system was simply too damaged. Stacey's treatment took 15 sessions over two years and incorporated several modalities including hypnosis, ego-state work, EMDR and somatic focused work.

The process consisted of 3 steps: 1) Understanding pain 2) Repairing mind-body reconnection and 3) Trauma processing/brain retraining. At the end of that time Stacey was largely free of pain, off all medication and working again. Her marriage had improved because of her learning to ask for what she wanted and share the load more with her husband, who fortunately was able to respond to her changes positively.

Neuro optometry

Specialist entry by Brenton Clark, neuro optometrist

Katie: How Brenton Clark changed my life.
When I saw Brenton, he was the first person that asked me
'Why do you want to get better?' This gave me intense focus,
but the introduction of prism/tinted glasses was a major
breakthrough in my recovery. The eyes are normally impacted
during a concussion, and investigating neuro optometry can be
a life-changing experience.

My name is Brenton Clark and I have been practising as a registered optometrist in New Zealand (with a few years in Australia) for more than 30 years. About 15 years ago, a client presented one day as a referral from her doctor. She was experiencing several visual difficulties since a concussion which had occurred a few months earlier and her doctor thought I'd be able to assist her. She was obviously suffering, yet my optometric examination did not reveal anything unusual about her eyes to account for her symptoms. It was a puzzle to me.

It was then that I remembered attending a seminar hosted by the Australasian College of Behavioural Optometry (ACBO) a few years previously on the topic of *acquired brain injury* and optometric management. At the time I thought the seminar was interesting but as I had never encountered anyone fitting this description, the information wasn't relevant. But now here in my examination chair was someone with a *brain injury*.

Revising the information presented at the seminar, I was able to assist this first client using a combination of tinted lenses and optometric vision therapy. She worked hard on the latter, and we achieved very pleasing results. It was not long afterwards that another client arrived in my examination room, also distressed, with a very similar profile of symptoms to the first client. And then another . . .

These days seeing several clients per week with persisting visual symptoms because of a concussion is commonplace.

Looking back, I realise the doctor who originally made the referral must have realised that an optometrist would be the logical choice for a client with (by this time) longstanding visual symptoms directly attributable to her concussion. Referral to an eye specialist (ophthalmologist) would be of far less value as he realised that no direct trauma to the eye had occurred. As professionals, we all have our own tools in our kitbag that we use. The tools in the kitbag of an ophthalmologist consist of medications (internal or topical) and/or surgery to the eye or lids.

The tools in the kitbag of a neuro optometrist are quite different and include optical lenses, prisms, chromatic filters (tints), selective occlusion, optometric light therapy (syntonics) and optometric vision therapy (sometimes erroneously referred to as 'eye exercises').

After seeing hundreds of clients over the years, it is very rare that I see any direct eye trauma associated with a traumatic brain injury. Signs of eye disease are sometimes noted and occasionally are contributory to symptoms, but by far most clients have multiple visual symptoms in the presence of healthy eyes. This all makes sense *considering it is the brain (not the eyes) which has suffered the injury*, as I shall attempt to explain.

The brain and vision

While visual acuity (clarity of sight) is one aspect of visual function, it is merely the tip of the iceberg, the result of just one of multiple processes which underly visual function. Vision is much more than how *clearly* we see, it is a dynamic interactive process of motor and sensory function, mediated by the eyes for the purpose of simultaneous organisation of posture, movement, spatial orientation, interaction with (and manipulation of) the environment, perception and thought.

Vision is our dominant sense. *70 per cent of the total sensory input to the brain comes from the eyes.* Two-thirds of the brain's electrical activity and half of the brain's cortex is involved in processing visual information. Accommodation, vergences, saccades, orbital sensation, eyelid function, visual fields, acuity, colour vision and pupillary function are subserved by 7 of the 12 cranial nerves. At least 32 different areas of the brain (including brainstem, subcortical, cerebellar and limbic areas) are recognised in the processing of visual information and at least 300 intracortical connecting pathways have been identified.

With such a complex network it should be clear that our sense of vision does not reside in any one area of the brain and most certainly does not reside in the eyeball itself. It should come as no surprise that any insult to the brain (including a mild traumatic brain injury such as concussion) is highly likely to disrupt one or more of these pathways and thereby affect visual function in some way. In the case of concussion, this could be due to the diffuse axonal injury (lasting hours to days) from the rapid acceleration/deceleration and shearing forces applied to the brain, or from the secondary inflammation and dysfunctional healing which can cause symptoms lasting for months or sometimes years.

Persistent low grade headache, post-traumatic migraine, disturbances to sleep, dizziness, nausea, light sensitivity, noise sensitivity, motion sensitivity (which together make visiting supermarket or shopping centre intolerable), blurred/ghosting/double vision, fatigue, concentration and memory difficulties and low tolerance to viewing screens are all typical post-concussion symptoms which can persist way beyond the usual time course for resolution of symptoms (which is usually 2-3 weeks for adults).

It is not known why a minority of individuals who suffer a concussion have symptoms which then persist for months or years, but certain risk factors have been identified. The time from diagnosis to receiving specialised concussion services, pre-existing mood disorders, having had one or more prior concussions, a history of migraines, dizziness at the time of the injury, being female – these are all some of the factors which may increase the risk of concussion symptoms persisting much longer than a few weeks.

For those suffering from such symptoms, the skills of a multi-disciplinary team are usually required. When there are persisting visual symptoms, one of the team members should be a neuro optometrist, an optometrist who has the necessary post-graduate training and experience to utilise the (almost) unique tools of the profession of optometry.

Neuro optometrists recognise that part of the concussion process (and subsequent characteristic symptoms) is caused by a disruption to at least two modes of visual processing which normally work harmoniously together. The neuroanatomy is complex, and much of the understanding has been determined by examining non-human primates, but there is no evidence to suggest the fundamentals are any different in humans.

One of the pathways, which neuro optometrists usually refer to as the 'focal' process (or ventral stream), involves so-called P (for parvocellular) fibres which arise from cells of the central retina. They connect to the lateral geniculate nucleus (a kind of relay station in the centre of the brain) and then the primary visual (occipital) cortex, the rear-most cortex of the brain. From here, fibres travel back to the LGN and the temporal cortex, influenced by areas of the brain responsible for attention, working memory and stimulus salience. The pathway forward towards the frontal lobe takes a lower route, giving the ventral stream its name. P fibres make up most fibres and are more sensitive to detail and colour and require more time (and light) to process attributes such as shape and form. The ventral processing stream is often referred to as the 'What' system as it answers the question 'What am I looking at?' (Reading an eye chart is a good example of the focal/ventral 'what' system at work).

A minority of fibres (called magnocellular or M fibres) arise from the peripheral retina of the eye and will eventually form the 'ambient' process (or dorsal stream). M fibres are sensitive to spatial location, orientation, change and movement so are fast acting in their response. They connect to the superior colliculus in the mid brain before moving on to connect to an area of the visual cortex called the middle temporal visual area (abbreviated as MT). Importantly, at the superior colliculus visual information is also integrated with auditory, proprioceptive, vestibular and cerebellar information from other sensory pathways.

There are two-way connections between MT and the superior colliculus, but MT primarily connects with the parietal cortex (located above the temporal cortex, hence the term 'dorsal' stream). From the parietal cortex, the dorsal stream breaks into further pathways moving forwards to the frontal cortex. Each sub-pathway mediates different aspects of visuospatial function.

The complex ambient network continually adjusts to the constant stream of sensory-motor input it is receiving and is therefore able to anticipate change pre-consciously. The ambient system can be regarded as the system which provides 'Where' information (as in 'Where am I and where is it in relation to me?') and plays a role in posture and balance.

The ambient system develops earlier and functions at a more subconscious level of awareness compared to the focal system which operates at a more conscious level. The focal system tends to work in isolation and is innate. As the ambient system integrates with other sensory systems it is largely learned and thus can be enhanced with training and rehabilitation. You could think of the ambient process as a grounding process, providing a stable platform within which the focal system can operate.

However, neither the ambient or focal processes operate in isolation from the other or with the rest of the body. Instead they work in a synergistic manner and as individuals we will all have our unique style of using these processes together. However, the dorsal location of the parietal cortex and greater complexity of pathways in this system also make it more vulnerable to disruption in a brain injury, in which case the characteristic symptoms seen in post-concussion syndrome arise.

Individuals who have suffered a concussion are often perplexed when they walk through a doorway only to find themselves banging their shoulder or reach for a glass and knock it over. How is this possible? It is easily explained by dysfunction of ambient processing which did not provide fast and accurate (pre-conscious) spatial information as to exactly where in space their moving body was located relative to the door (or where their moving hand was located relative to the glass).

How things are to be done require accurate spatial ('Where is it relative to me?') information to be processed. Visual implications of ambient/dorsal stream dysfunction include:

- Problems with eye teaming control (such as poor convergence)
- Problems with eye movements (such as saccades and pursuits)
- Problems with spatial awareness
- Problems with accommodation (focusing) control
- Problems with visual-vestibular functioning
- Problems with reaction time
- Problems with executive functioning

When the ambient system is not functioning properly and there is no automatic anticipation, the individual finds themself always on the back foot, in a reacting mode. Not only is this more fatiguing but anxiety levels are likely to increase, for what should be simple everyday actions now require far more concentration and care to accomplish.

Other common symptoms such as light and motion sensitivity can be hypothesised by ambient dysfunction as M cells are much more sensitive to luminance contrast than P cells, and M cells as part of the dorsal processing stream converge to regions of the brain (such as the middle temporal visual area) which detect and process motion.

Optometric tools in concussion injury

The following tools are available to the neuro optometrist. Most will in some way adjust the focal-ambient dynamic in such a way as to reduce symptoms, increase function and thus assist with overall rehabilitation.

Concussion glasses may incorporate one or more of the following;

- Bi-nasal occlusion
- Selective chromatic filters (tints)
- Prism (base-in microprism or yoked prism)
- Selective occlusion or spot occlusion
- Lenses, especially low plus lenses

Other neuro optometric treatments include

- Syntonic light therapy
- Optometric vision therapy

Some tools are a passive treatment in that the lens, prism or chromatic filter effects the change. Other tools (such as optometric vision therapy) require active engagement and effort to effect the desired changes in function. There is no risk with appropriately and carefully prescribed concussion glasses, and they are often very effective in helping to reduce symptoms and improve the effectiveness of rehabilitation therapies. However, there is usually no circumstance where concussion glasses alone effect a recovery from post-concussion syndrome. They are just one tool (albeit a useful tool) to assist with rehabilitation.

Specific chromatic filters and concussion

Extreme sensitivity to light (photophobia) is so common following a traumatic brain injury that clients will often be seen wearing sunglasses (and a cap or brimmed hat) as they sit awaiting their appointment. The light sensitivity is such that normal indoor lighting (especially fluorescent lighting), looking at screens and any examination techniques involving localised illumination can cause significant discomfort.

The sensitivity not only limits activities and quality of life but may trigger or exacerbate a headache. When lights cannot be avoided, the discomfort can persist long after exposure to the light source. Relatively constant photophobia at a patient's workplace or in a classroom may be a contributing factor to end of day fatigue, headache and other symptoms.

Although the use of sunglasses inside is *effective*, it is not recommended if you can get specific chromatic filter tints. Traditional sunglasses usually diminish all frequencies of light and decrease contrast, making visual observations indoors difficult and impracticable.

Specific chromatic filters (tints) are superior to sunglass wear inside as they mitigate photosensitivity and can reduce post-traumatic headaches, motion sensitivity and 'dry eye' ocular discomfort while still maintaining contrast and detail of sensory information. Firstly, they are not as dark (usually in the 15 to 40 per cent absorbance range) and are frequency specific to the individual.

A mismatched tint colour will likely not provide the immense relief so often noted, even though the tint is still absorbing some degree of light. I have found that almost all symptomatic clients will benefit immediately (and often profoundly) from a chromatic filter – it is just a matter of finding the most effective one. Comments are usually along the lines of 'My brain seems calmer', 'Everything looks clearer', 'The carpet pattern isn't moving now', along with the obvious 'It's not so bright now'. While the colour of the tint can vary from client to client, I have personally found the most commonly effective chromatic filter is 30 per cent blue, followed by 30 per cent amber and FL41 (a light plum colour) of similar absorbance. I have also found that when blue is preferred indoors, then dark grey (polarised) is the most effective sunglass colour for outdoor wear. Conversely, if amber (or FL41) is the preferred indoor chromatic filter, then dark brown (polarised) is often the sunglass colour to recommend. Ideally, clients should have a chance to trial a specific tint colour over a few days or more to establish the potential benefit of the proposed chromatic filter.

Visual Motion Sensitivity (VMS) and concussion

Visual Motion Sensitivity is a condition where nausea, dizziness and possible loss of balance occurs when moving in certain situations and/or when surroundings are moving in one's peripheral vision. Concussion or other head injuries (and some neurological conditions) are the main cause of VMS. Symptoms may be reported with many of the following:

- Watching or scrolling lines on a computer screen

- Walking in busy shopping centres or in supermarket aisles
- Sitting in the passenger or back seat of a moving car
- Riding on an escalator
- Inability to comfortably wear multifocal (progressive) spectacle lenses
- Watching action movies (or quick changes of scene), especially when seated close to the screen
- Inability to use virtual reality headsets.

As discussed, VMS results from dysfunction of ambient processing – the visual system is having difficulty quickly and accurately processing movement of surrounding vision. VMS often accompanies pattern glare (an intolerance to carpet or clothing patterns) and light sensitivity.

The following therapies may help reduce the symptoms associated with VMS: Selective chromatic filters (tints), especially if pattern glare is also present, bi-nasal occlusion, small amounts of base-in prism, neuro-optometric vision therapy to develop normal eye movements, better integrate focal and ambient visual processing, and improve visual-vestibular function.

Dry eye and concussion

Dry eye symptoms include dry, scratchy and gritty discomfort, or ocular pain sensations (which may be spontaneous or evoked by wind or light). A known reality of dry eye is that the surface signs observed often corelate poorly with the severity of symptoms. This suggests that factors beyond localised tear film and ocular health are driving the ocular pain symptoms. Indeed, dry eye, migraine and photophobia are a common triad of symptoms associated with a brain injury.

A trigeminal nerve dysfunction in peripheral and central nerves connecting the cornea to the brain is hypothesised as the source of this greater-than-expected level of pain, with similar mechanisms also accounting for the pain and photophobia associated with the brain injury. Treatment of dry eye with traditional recommendations (ocular lubricants and lid hygiene protocols, especially when there are lid signs of meibomian gland dysfunction) is recommended but may not be totally effective without addressing the nerve pathways. Chromatic filters, for example, will often help decrease dry eye ocular pain (along with the corresponding migraine and photophobia).

Progressive lenses and concussion

Progressive lenses, also known as PALs (progressive addition lenses), multifocals or varifocals are a common type of lens worn by adults over the age 45 years with presbyopia. (Presbyopia occurs when the crystalline lens within the eye is unable to change focus from distance to near – this means holding print back further away from the eyes or using stronger glasses for reading).

If one looks around the room wearing reading glasses, everything will appear blurry. Progressive lenses allow for clear distance vision (looking through the upper part of the lens) and reading (looking through the lower part of the lens) and are very popular due to the convenience of having just one pair of glasses for all tasks.

If you are suffering from post-concussion symptoms and wear progressive lenses, it is more likely than not that they will at best <u>slow</u> your recovery and at worst <u>prolong</u> your recovery, even if prior to the brain injury you were able to tolerate progressive glasses without any difficulties.

This is because these lenses induce subtle distortions in the peripheral zones of the lens which all wearers must adapt to. As we have discussed, it is often the case that following a brain injury, spatial vision (i.e., ambient visual processing) is altered and the peripheral lens distortions induced by progressive lenses serve to multiply this peripheral disturbance effect on spatial vision.

The possible consequences include disequilibrium, dizziness, spatial insecurity and visual fatigue or eye discomfort. If you typically wear progressive lenses, what happens when you read with single focus lenses? Depending on your individual prescription, your eyes may be suitable for readymade ('hobby') glasses. If you don't have poor unaided general (distance) vision, what happens to symptoms when you move around with progressive glasses removed? For similar reasons, multifocal contact lenses or monovision/blended wear contact lenses could also be more symptom provoking than single focus distance contact lenses.

Bi-nasal Occlusion (BNO) and concussion

Bi-nasal occlusion is a method of partially occluding part of the nasal visual field in each eye by means of opaque or semi-opaque tape applied to glasses. This can be a client's own existing glasses or sunglasses, or (if the client doesn't wear glasses) plano computer glasses can be used to support the BNO tape. In some cases, the effects of bi-nasal occlusion on symptoms can be significant. (Others might note only a small benefit, and some not at all).

How does occluding a small area of visual field work? There are various hypotheses for the mechanism of action, but changing the visual input in some way provides the brain with an opportunity to process visual information differently. Perhaps reducing the amount of overlap in vision from each eye reduces 'visual background noise', or perhaps the relationship between focal and ambient processing of vision is altered.

In any case, BNO appears to be especially effective in helping severe visual spatial symptoms such as visual motion sensitivity, headache, nausea, vertigo and balance issues. Give it a try if you have any of these symptoms. The advantage of BNO is that it is simple and available to all – you just need some opaque tape or semi-opaque scotch tape.

Materials required:

1) Glasses. Your own or hobby specs (if not a suitable strength, remove the

    lenses) or plano blue filter computer glasses

2) Opaque scotch tape or similar

The steps:

1) If for reading: read something aloud without the tape on the glasses. If for general wear, move around in a small figure of eight path, moving your head and eyes around.

2) Apply tape to the glasses over the inner nasal area of the lens – do each side symmetrically. Usually the tape is angled inwards a little, but you can also try vertically – one might be noticeably better than the other.

3) Try reading as before. Is it easier to read? (*Faster or words appear more stable or clearer?*) Try walking around as before. Is there anything noticeably easier? (*Less dizzy, feeling more balanced, objects in room appear more stationary?*)

4) If not, peel the tape off and move it further outwards by just a millimetre on each side, then try step 3 again.

5) Repeat as many times as necessary with the tape being attached further and further outward by small increments. If

the tape is now so far across your vision that it is distracting and annoying, then you have gone too far. If you have not noted any improvement for better by this stage, then BNO might not be of use to you.

The Brain Injury Symptom Survey

The Brain Injury Vision Symptom Survey (BIVSS) is a great tool in common use which highlights (to both patient and professionals alike) how vision may have been altered because of an acquired brain injury. Score the questionnaire after completion; more than 30 points is significant, and a neuro-optometric assessment is likely to be of benefit. Here is a copy of the BIVSS:

SYMPTOM / BEHAVIOUR HOW OFTEN DO YOU CURRENTLY EXPERIENCE ANY OF THE FOLLOWING. (CIRCLE A NUMBER)	Never	Seldom	Occasionally	Frequently	Always	Prior to Injury?	Score Freq 1-4
EYESIGHT CLARITY							
Distance Vision Blurred – even with corrective lenses	0	1	2	3	4	☐	
Near Vision Blurred – even with corrective lenses	0	1	2	3	4	☐	
Clarity of vision changes / fluctuates during the day	0	1	2	3	4	☐	
Poor night vision / cannot see to drive at night	0	1	2	3	4	☐	
EYE TEAMING/ BINOCULAR VISION							
Double vision	0	1	2	3	4	☐	
Close or covers an eye to see clearly	0	1	2	3	4	☐	
Print moves in and out of focus when reading	0	1	2	3	4	☐	
VISION COMFORT							
Eye discomfort / sore eyes / eyestrain	0	1	2	3	4	☐	
Headaches or dizziness after using eyes	0	1	2	3	4	☐	
"Pulling" feeling around eyes	0	1	2	3	4	☐	
Eye fatigue / tired after using eyes	0	1	2	3	4	☐	
LIGHT SENSITIVITY							
Normal indoor lighting is uncomfortable / glary	0	1	2	3	4	☐	
Outdoor lighting is too bright – must use sunglasses	0	1	2	3	4	☐	
Fluorescent lighting is bothersome	0	1	2	3	4	☐	
DRY EYES							
Eyes feel "dry" / scratchy / sting	0	1	2	3	4	☐	
"Stare" into space without blinking	0	1	2	3	4	☐	
Rub eyes a lot	0	1	2	3	4	☐	
DEPTH PERCEPTION							
Misjudge where objects really are / Clumsiness	0	1	2	3	4	☐	
Lack of confidence walking / missing steps / stumbling	0	1	2	3	4	☐	
Poor hand writing (spacing, size, legibility)	0	1	2	3	4	☐	
PERIPHERAL VISION							
Avoid crowds / cannot tolerate busy places	0	1	2	3	4	☐	
What looks straight ahead is not always straight ahead	0	1	2	3	4	☐	
Side vision different / objects move or change position	0	1	2	3	4	☐	
READING							
Short attention span / easily distracted when reading	0	1	2	3	4	☐	
Difficulty / slowed reading or writing	0	1	2	3	4	☐	
Poor comprehension / cannot recall what was read	0	1	2	3	4	☐	
Confusion of words / skip words while reading	0	1	2	3	4	☐	
Loss of place /use finger too keep place when reading	0	1	2	3	4	☐	
Totals							
Cumulative Total							

Conclusion

If you are experiencing the range of typical symptoms associated with concussion (such as difficulties focussing, (usually variable) blurred or ghosting or double vision, light sensitivity, dizziness, nausea, headaches, fatigue or aching eyes and your eye professional tells you 'There is nothing wrong with your vision', then seek assistance elsewhere for you know yourself there most definitely is something wrong with your vision!

If your eye care professional tells you 'There is nothing wrong with your eyes' but they have no suggestions to help with your visual symptoms then again *seek assistance elsewhere*, for while it is reassuring that your eyes are healthy, it is apparent this professional does not have the specialised knowledge to assist you.

Both the focal and ambient visual processes must be assessed – the latter will usually require some assessment, which requires you to stand up out of the examination chair and move in real space.

Alternative eye therapies for concussion

Specialist entry: by Bradley Pillay (neurodevelopmental optometrist)

Katie: How Bradley Pillay changed my life:
I met Bradley through working with a remote client online who had recently suffered concussion. After suggesting the client's mother contact her local neuro optometrist, she told me of the new technology Bradley was using to help her brain. Technology is advancing in so many ways that it is important to research the new modalities to help your brain.

As an optometrist for over 15 years my practice has focused on a neuro-developmental approach to visual processing. I have always been fascinated with the brain and found my knowledge around its function and action lacking when I started practising as an optometrist.

Over time, I have found a distinct similarity between the visual presentation of a neurodiverse individual and those who had experienced traumatic brain injuries or acquired brain injuries. We have only had training as part of our degree that I now consider very basic. Most general optometrists will only ever consider physical structural abnormalities, pathology or optical issues in these cases, which woefully misses the real reason behind individuals experiencing their issues which is an imbalance in the autonomic nervous system due to their trauma response and overactivation of the sympathetic pathways. Although correcting their prescription requirements with their spectacle or prismatic needs could help some of their symptoms.

It does not fully answer all the difficulties they present with. Initially, whilst finding my feet as an optometrist, *I did what every other practitioner did and continued repeating 'These things take time to heal'*. Unfortunately, this blanket response was all I could offer my patients at the time. I had no concrete answers which annoyed my need to 'Fix their problem' – which is where my journey to becoming a neurodevelopmental optometrist and exploring neuro optometric rehabilitation methods really started.

Through continued exploration of many different disciplines, I started to build an understanding of what happens when things in the body go wrong with trauma and how the visual system mirrors these responses, the pattern of responses being what I describe as *sympathetic overstimulation*. I began to see that our understanding of the autonomic nervous system is essential to understanding the reactions (or over-reactions) found when we assess our patient.

With concussion, be it TBI or ABI, we are fortunate if we know when the traumatic event took place and the way it took place. Regardless, the visual system will almost always respond in the same way if we are careful to observe how an individual processes space. It is also very important to note that the visual system never reacts in isolation.

The autonomic nervous system (ANS), endocrine and limbic systems will also be influenced by the trauma, at least in part. This does depend on how long the reaction from the trauma is sustained. A neurological reaction that lasts more than two weeks is considered chronic and capable of stalling or deregulating neurological systems.

How do we process space? (width, depth and height)

Our optical prescription could be thought of essentially as the focus of the eye – how far can I see (mostly central vision). The width and height of our visual space is related to our visual attention to that space. I.e., what is the body allowing the visual system to be processed? Attention is the ability to attend to something.

In sensory attention, our ability to do something is related to how much the body is allowing it to be processed. In other words, if the body is busy doing something else such as healing or fighting off an infection, it cannot allow full attention on most of the sensory systems to process information in its fullness. In neurological terms, this is the balance of the autonomic nervous system (the balance between parasympathetic and sympathetic pathways).

A full neurodevelopmental or behavioural optometric assessment is recommended for anyone who has experienced TBI/ABI or presents with suspected or diagnosed specific learning or specific behavioural patterns. Interpretation of the findings can and will give us a visual system response that mirrors the balance of the ANS (autonomic nervous system) if we carefully analyse the findings. In addition to this, plotting our functional kinetic colour visual fields is essential to understanding how the visual pathways are being affected by the balance of the ANS.

Colour visual fields

This is a measurement of the functional visual fields of the eyes. The physical visual field is a measure of how much peripheral vision a person has and is dependent on the health of the person's visual system, retina and brain. This is affected by sinister events such as brain tumours, strokes, cataracts and/or retinal disease.

The functional visual field is a measure of how much of the physical visual field the visual system can process and concentrate on. This field is a dynamic field and can change and vary depending on the state of the person's autonomic nervous system. If the fields are found to be reduced or out of balance, this means their ANS is out of balance. We are often able to increase their size during vision training activities when we incorporate optometric photo biomodulation into the activities.

The autonomic nervous system is made up of two parts – the parasympathetic system and the sympathetic system. These systems are naturally antagonistic. Any long-term disruption of the balance can affect our colour visual fields and cause constrictions in them. If your colour visual fields are normal it is usually an indication of a normal functional ocular system and a fully functioning and balanced autonomic nervous system.

All sensory receptors in our body respond to stimuli only if the autonomic nervous system allows it. i.e., our retinal photo receptors will only be attentive to information if the autonomic nervous system allows it and is in some form of balance. Automated visual fields are used in optometry to measure and detect departures from normal, which is indicative of pathology.

Colour visual fields are measurements taken through the visual system and represent the total sensory input, integration and output response of the individual to a visual stimulus. When there is interference in the neural flow of input-process-output, a reduced response is given.

The individual's sensitivity, awareness, understanding and response are reduced, resulting in a reduced colour visual field. Improvements in the functional visual field size forms a tracking system to show whether our training is working or not. We all have inherited an autonomic nervous system from our parents that would either be in perfect balance, sympathetically dominant or para-sympathetically dominant.

This internal, genetically determined response system reacts to stimuli depending on what the body requires. Our sympathetic system predominates while we are awake (fight or flight system, adrenal system) and our para-sympathetic system predominates while we are asleep (rest and digest system, healing, sleep). External events such as trauma (be it physical, emotional, real or perceived) can result in our autonomic nervous system reacting. These reactions can sometimes cause cortical and sub-cortical 'reaction memories' associated with the nervous system that 'pre-programme' the nervous system to react a certain way to trauma, infection, etc.

Optometric photobiomodulation (syntonics)

To determine if there is an imbalance in the autonomic nervous system we perform a baseline colour visual fields test, which is a measurement of the functional visual fields of the eyes. The functional visual field is a measure of how much physical visual field the visual system can concentrate on and process.

This field is a dynamic field and can vary depending on the state of the person's autonomic nervous system. When our sympathetic system is stuck in 'on' mode our ocular functions can break down (accommodation, convergence, 3D vision and fusion). Any long-term disruption of the balance of the nervous system can affect the colour visual fields and cause constrictions in them.

Light pathways explanation:

Light is processed via three main pathways in our body through our eyes. (Light can also be processed through our skin whereby our skin produces Vitamin D from exposure to UV B light). Two pathways are for sight (seeing pathways) and one is for regulation of our autonomic nervous system via the thalamus and hypothalamus (non-seeing pathways). Our seeing pathways are made up of magnocellular and parvocellular pathways which take information from our rods and cones.

The magnocellular pathways allow processing of brightness, high contrast, movement, 3D vision, whereas the parvocellular pathways allow processing of colour, high resolution. The magnocellular gives us an idea of 'Where is it?' and the parvocellular gives us an idea of 'What is it?' Both the 'where' and the 'what' need to be working together and integrated together to have a fully functional visual system.

Balancing of the nervous system is achieved through expanding the functional visual fields by stimulating the retina with specific frequencies of light in the form of special layered filters that allow exposure to these frequencies for 20 minutes, 2x a day for 6-10 weeks (performed at home). By doing this, we can boost the electrical signal between the receptors on the retina and the visual system (as if we were turning the volume up). We then re-measure the functional visual fields to ensure progress and adjust the frequencies if necessary.

Depending on how restricted the field is to begin with, expansion may take 3-6 weeks and sometimes require an additional stimulation in this same way 3-6 months later. My preference in concussion rehab is to stabilise the primary sense (visual system) and the hypothalamic responses. This allows the body to be more responsive to therapy and training where we are trying to create either new patterns of movement/behaviour or trying to connect with available but suppressed patterns of movement/behaviour. All of this is in an attempt to achieve automaticity and smoother processing of either movement or sensory information.

Once the visual system is stabilised, my preference at this point is to introduce physical activity to integrate the visual sensory system together with the motor system and vestibular system with free-space exercises for both the eyes and the vestibular system (co-ordination and balance). Although computer-based vision therapy can be beneficial, many patients I am dealing with have a high level of light sensitivity and visual stress. Therapy on a computer could potentially exacerbate their visual stress.

Our aim is to facilitate sensory integration through multisensory stimulation. When you stimulate the senses simultaneously, we facilitate integration and hopefully a visual system that functions better overall. The final visual training may take 2-3+ months at home with reviews approximately monthly depending on progress.

Visual stress

Visual stress is a condition that is best described as a visual processing disorder where someone experiences distortion or visual disturbances when looking at high contrast information such as text. They would often see movement, colours, flickering, waving, flashing or even observe words disappear off the page while reading.

This leads to slower reading and comprehension. This is caused by a disruption and overload of their neurological pathways. These individuals often suffer from sensory processing overload – i.e. they experience issues with other senses, such as discomfort or increased distraction with a loud or noisy environment or pickiness with touch or tastes. This overload causes poor concentration and reduces cognitive function.

To understand, from a neurological point of view, what is happening in their brain we first must describe what we know about how a neuron transmits information through different pathways.

Firstly, let's briefly explain communication theory. In any signal-based system – i.e. all our senses, radio and television transmission, telecommunications, etc – information is passed through the network as 'signal'. There is also always noise in this system. The signal must be powerful and clear enough to overcome the noise and to be received and interpreted. Let's just put that explanation aside for now.

A neuron in the visual system is stimulated by a flash of light, yet we see that before a flash is received the neuron has a background (resting) electrical activity. A single flash that is received causes the neuron to get excited and electrical activity sharply rises then gradually falls. This is mediated by neurotransmitters – little chemicals that stimulate the neurons to excitement.

A normal neuron will then return to rest after a period which we label as 't'. If we looked at an immature neuron, such as what we find in the pathways of those with learning disabilities and visual stress, *we find that their return to rest is much longer than normal.* If we fired two flashes of light you can see that a normal neuron is ready to receive and process the information whereas the immature neuron is already excited and will just go into overload due to delayed recovery.

Let's put this into perspective for what a child may see. A child will look at a word on a high contrast page. Each edge of the letter can be thought of as tiny flashes of light to the brain (an increase in brightness of the light on the page). The very thing we are trying to get the child to read causes an overload to their visual system, resulting in poor concentration, reading speed, tracking, comprehension, etc.

They may also have reduced visual acuity as a result but – important to mention – this may not be a glasses issue but a neural pathway issue. Many children would look at a word and the word would remain imprinted in their visual system – when they look at another word on the page the result is an overlap of the words, leading to more visual confusion. So in terms of communication theory the resulting visual distortion – 'noise' – overrides the signal 'text', resulting in a breakdown of comfortable reading.

Why do children see these distortions such as coloured spots, waves, rivers, flickering, patterns, etc? Are they lying? Well, the neurons that are being overloaded only know how to process light, so when their processing is overloaded, it will show as light and visual distortions.

The best way to imagine what they see is like listening to a radio that has not been properly tuned – static is what *you hear*, distortions is what *they see*. What do we do about this? We first identify what part of the spectrum, if any, is causing this disruption. The cause. This is done through a series of questions with visual tasks and coloured overlays. If they show benefit from the use of an overlay, then we treat it with coloured filters often in the form of coloured spectacles.

Visual stress could be a large cause of the issues but an evaluation through a screening process would be recommended.

Self-help eye exercises

Specialist entry: by Ryan O'Connor Neuro optometrist

Saccades are eye movements that *quickly shift the eye's focus between two fixed points*. We use them when driving, we use them when reading – every eye movement that involves scanning our environment is a saccade.

Healthy brains do this quickly. However, brain injuries and damaged neural pathways can lead to irregular eye movements.

This is caused by the narrowing of the visual system due to the dominance of the brain stem. The visual system needs to open again and integrate the periphery, which it needs to do for proper eye movement and proper integration with the vestibular system.

When moving the eyes from side to side, or up and down, or point to point on the clock face, become aware of the point you are jumping to within your periphery, prior to activating the eye movement.

So the eye exercises that you are given to rehabilitate are very important. If you haven't been given eye exercises, here are some basic ones to get you started. I would recommend (if you are working with a physiotherapist) to get a specialist to guide you through these. With these exercises ONLY GO TO THE POINT OF NAUSEA and then stop. Consistency is always more important than quantity.

Peripheral integration exercise

When sitting on the toilet use the door frame to open the vision up:

1. Stare at the door handle
2. While staring at the door handle, visualise the top right corner in your periphery
3. Point with your arm at the top right corner, then move your eyes.
4. Next repeat with the top left corner, then the bottom left, bottom right and back to the door handle.

The modified Brock's String

This can be done anywhere using the index finger from each hand;

1. Bring your index finger as close as you can focus then move it back ever so slightly and focus on your fingerprints.
2. Place the index finger of your other hand directly behind your first hand about 150mm behind.
3. Stay focussed on your front fingerprint and you should be able to see a double image of your back finger.
4. Now jump your fixation to the back finger and focus on your fingerprint there.
5. You should now see the front finger as a double image.
6. Jump back and forth 20 times each day.

A video from Insight vision optometry:

https://www.youtube.com/watch?v=4rDygaF3Dog

Jump ductions

1. Ensure you have your glasses on if you have a prescription. If you require both distance and near focus, wear the glasses prescribed to correct these.

2. Focus on a close target such as numbers on your phone or in a book and jump to a similar focal target across the room such as a clock face, maybe a digital clock on an oven/microwave/DVD player.

3. Bring the *near* task into focus (the book or phone), then jump the gaze to the far target (the clock).

4. When the far target (clock) is in focus return to the near target (book or phone), when it is in focus again return to the distance focus (clock).

5. Practice this 20 times.

References

- Daniel G. Amen MD, Tana Amen BSN, RN, *The Brain Warrior's Way*. Published by Penguin Books, 2018
- Mark D. Grant MA, *Change your brain, change your pain*. Published by Amazon, 2016
- Byron Katie, Stephen Mitchell, *Loving What Is*. Published by Penguin Books
- Sadhguru, *Inner Engineering: A Yogi's Guide to Joy*. Published by Harmony/Rodale
- Daniel G. Amen, MD, Tana Amen BSN, RN, *The Brain Warrior's Way Cookbook*. Published by Penguin Books
- Mike Dow MD, *The Brain Fog Fix*. Published by Hay House, 2015
- Leah Hectman, *Clinical Naturopathic Medicine*. Published by Elsevier, 2012
- Pete Egoscue, *Pain Free, A Revolutionary Method for Stopping Chronic Pain*. Published by Bantam, 1998
- Louise L. Hay, *You Can Heal Your Life*. Published by Hay House
- Gary Chapman, *The 5 Love Languages: The Secret to Love that Lasts*. Published by Moody
- Marilyn Light, *Hypoglycaemia*. Published by McGraw Hill (Good Health Guide Series)
- Dr Paavo Airola, *Hypoglycaemia: A Better Approach*. Published by Health Plus Publishers
- Mark Grant MA, 'Overcoming Pain' website. https://overcomingpain.com/
- www.headway.org.nz
- Complete Concussion Management Inc (CCMI), Dr Cameron Marshall. www.completeconcussions.com

- ACC. www.acc.co.nz
- Huberman Lab. www.hubermanlab.com
- Brain Injury Association USA https://biausa.org/
- Brain injury UK https://www.headway.org.uk/
- Brain injury NZ https://brain-injury.nz/
- Brain Injury Canada https://braininjurycanada.ca/en/
- If you want to learn more about the brain go to www.amenuniversity.com
- If you are looking for an optometrist with the required knowledge and skills to effectively help visual symptoms which have occurred because of an acquired brain injury, then the ACBO and NORA websites are a great resource. www.acbo.org.au
  www.noravisionrehab.org

About Katie Jolly

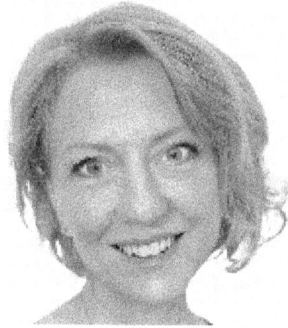

Katie Jolly lives with her husband and two children in New Zealand. Katie is a natural health practitioner, author, brain health educator, public speaker, and an advocate for mental (brain) health.

She is a licensed Elite Brain Health Trainer through the Amen University and passionate about helping others navigate brain health.

She believes that, just like nature, healing takes time and patience, but growth always happens—even in the dirt.

You can connect with Katie here: www.katiejollynd.com

www.ingramcontent.com/pod-product-compliance
Lightning Source LLC
Chambersburg PA
CBHW022330280326
41934CB00006B/586